I MISS YOU MOM

A Daughter's Journey Into Dementia Land

Faith Marshall

Contact the Author
Faith Marshall llc
12345 Lake City Way NE #260
Seattle, WA 98125

www.faithmarshall.com/staying-connected

info@faithmarshall.com

4

DEDICATION

I dedicate this book to Dennis, my oldest brother. With his unconditional love and care, Dennis dedicated his precious time, vast management skills and talents to managing both Dad's and Mom's care. He coordinated appointments, home repairs, in-home care staff, treatments, medications, care plans, facility tours and kept family all on the same page via emails, phone calls and family meetings. Each step of the way, with a smile on his face and a lot of miles on those tires, ferry rides, tolls and whatever it took. When he asked for our support or needed something, Rick and I honored his heartfelt and well planned requests. His commute to Seattle was over 2 hours each way and that did not keep him from often traveling several times a week. He did not know that he was battling cancer, nor could we anticipate the possibility that it would take him from us almost one year to the day after Mom passed away. Bless you, dearest Bro. I think I hear your music playing from heaven.

<u>ACKNOWLEDGEMENTS</u>

To my editor, awarding-winning author and fine friend, J. R. Nakken: With a loving heart you encouraged me, taught me, coached me, scolded me and praised my work. With much gratitude forever and more lunches to come.

To BJ, my sis-in-law and first editor, who painstakingly corrected my numerous bloopers in pen on paper with the artistry of a seasoned teacher. I will forever remember all your loving notes of encouragement. I love you!

To all the friends and family that took the time to proofread, comment, cry, laugh and encourage me. Rick, Lynne, Steve, Mary, Jan, Donna, Terry, Deetsy and Cathy, I appreciate all your help and support.

Last by certainly not least, I want to thank the management staff and legal teams from the homes where Mom lived, who read and granted approval and support for this book. A big shout out to the wonderful staff and caregivers that cared for Dad and Mom over the years. We were blessed to have you in our lives and learn from you. Thank you!

TABLE OF CONTENTS

INTRODUCTION

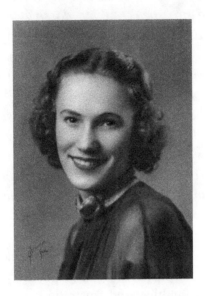

She looks in the mirror and the person looking back is much older; she may not even recognize the reflection. In her mind's eye is a much younger image of herself in the mirror; her children are younger, her mother is still alive and she most certainly has no grandchildren. The person in the room with her is just a familiar face, but she says she is her daughter, and is fifty years old; how can that be?

How did I get from there to here, she wonders? Did I just wake up from a dream and missed all the years in between? Why can't I say the words that I am trying to speak? Why doesn't this woman understand me? When I say, "I don't want to be here," and ask "How did I get here," she just says, "I know you don't but it's what is best for you," and, "we brought you here in the car." What in the world is she talking about? I don't understand how I got here! What on earth happened to my home, my car and where is my mother? My mother would never leave me here like this! Whose house is this anyway, and who are all these old people? How do they all know my name?

I write this story about my mom, Corrine, to share our family's experiences with memory loss, its oddities, difficulties, and frustrations as well as the amazement and regard for the human mind.

Watching a loved one change in any way is difficult. Mom's experience was with dementia, which presented as confusion and loss of memory. According to statistics, one in six of us will die from Alzheimer's or other types of dementia in our elder years. It is currently the sixth leading cause of death. This book is meant to provide comfort to you and those affected by the circumstances you and your loved one will face throughout the journey.

In my case, fear was paramount with each visit, always hoping that she still remembered me. I am grateful that she never forgot my face. Somehow, some way, Mom still maintained her quick wit, no matter the state of her confusion. Primarily, I would like to share stories that occurred as her dementia progressed over the course of six plus years.

I hope that these stories provide a sense of support and comfort for you. Although your experience is very personal, know that others have survived and, without a doubt, you will, too.

Your loved one might be your dad, your mom, your sister, brother, spouse or a dear friend. The overwhelming loss feels the same. I hope my story helps alleviate some of your fears and supplies you with the strength to enjoy the moments and humor that, when viewed with a smile and an open heart, can bless your journey together.

The 5th Avenue

Dressed in feathers, high heeled shoes with taps, fishnet stockings on legs that went on and on, she lined up and marched onto the stage behind the robust red velvet curtain. The announcer bellowed, "Please take your seats, the show is about to begin." The trumpets blared with *Broadway Baby*.

The curtain strained to glide open. Corrine, center stage, froze as she heard the troupe leader whisper, "5, 6, 7, 8." Her feet shuffled, searching for the right steps. Struggling to remember the dance, she counted to herself, wanted to catch up as she shuffled and dare not tap a sound to the wrong beat as she followed her partner to stage left. She was lost on the stage where she had performed with rhythmic perfection so many times before.

It was the dress rehearsal for opening night at the 5th Avenue Theater in Seattle. Corrine sat quietly, watching from backstage as her understudy took her place.

For five years she stuck to her story that she stopped dancing due to arthritis in her knees.

Forgetful in Phoenix

I had some timeshare points that I needed to use before they expired and invited Mom with me on a trip. She was concerned about leaving Dad, since he depended on her for meals and she was just as dependent upon their routines. I must admit, up to this point, the only forgetful symptoms that Mom had exhibited was the occasional repetition of a story or happening and forgetting that she had already told me. Sometimes this would occur within the same phone conversation. It was infrequent enough that it was not yet a significant concern. She occasionally confused time of day, and assuming she had just awakened from a nap, I would remind her that it was 8 p.m., not 8 a.m. when she mentioned she had to fix breakfast for Dad. My early response to these curiosities was the beginning of my own denial, justifying it by assuming the incidents were infrequent and therefore insignificant.

I made arrangements for Dad's care at home along with the flight arrangements and took the liberty of requesting wheelchair assistance, since Mom had such difficulty walking with her cane. She was not one to give up her independence, but cooperated with the wheelchair escort through the security station and straight to the gate. As a side benefit, I think she enjoyed all the personal attention. If you have not tried this, it is a courtesy of the airlines and simplifies travel through the airports and baggage claim on the co-travelers as well. It is difficult to rush an 89 year old woman with a cane and baggage through the security cattle chutes at the airport!

The flight was a non-stop to Phoenix, which also made our travel easier. We were greeted at the gate with another wheelchair escort to baggage claim and while the courtesy clerk waited with Mom, I checked out a rental car. We did the usual routine: rented the car, got baggage, wheeled Mom to the car and headed south with an hour's drive ahead of us. We talked along the way about the beautiful weather, the desert scenery and all the usual out of town observations.

Checking into the timeshare was standard procedure for me, but Mom became confused about where we were going when we got back in the car to follow the map and drive to the assigned condo. I had to explain to her several times that this was my unit, but I didn't own it as an individual unit. I don't think she ever understood the timeshare concept, but she loved its Southwestern decor and that she had her own private bedroom, as well as her own bathroom. We unpacked her bags and got all settled in. I wanted to go to the grocery store and get us some basics for the next few days' meals, so we headed back out the door, found where the closest local grocery store was and discussed the meals we would like to prepare.

She asked me, "Where did that nice girl go?"

"What nice girl?" Now I was confused.

She replied, "The one who picked us up at the airport."

I thought *This is strange* and said, "Mom, that was me!"

She was adamant. "No it wasn't, she drove so nicely and knew exactly where she was going!" She was so insistent, it was funny. Considering all that time riding right next to me in the front seat, I couldn't figure out how she could think I was someone else, but it made me laugh.

I just said, "Well, it was me. Sorry, Mom, but I had a map and I did know where I was going!"

Off we went shopping, and she had some very specific items she wanted to make sure I bought: a special kind of margarine and bread for her morning toast, etc. When we returned to the timeshare unit, we watched some TV, had dinner and got settled for bed. I made certain she had her book by her bedside as she was accustomed to reading when she woke up in the middle of the night.

The following morning, I wanted to go sit by the pool and take advantage of the warm sunshine. Of course, it took a while to get all our stuff together, pack snacks, beverages and drive over in the car, so that Mom didn't have to walk far. We parked in the handicapped space right next to the pool house entrance, unloaded all our gear and went outside to choose our spot near the pool. Mom stayed there, happily seated in the gazebo, while I ran inside to change into my swimsuit. When I returned, I pulled a chaise lounge into the sun, between the gazebo and the pool. Mom didn't want to be in the direct sunlight, but I did. I mentioned something about how nice the weather was and asked if she was comfortable. We chitchatted a bit, then I went into the pool and came back to dry off and sunbathe.

Mom was never one to sit silently, so we visited a little with various comments about the weather, the nice landscape, and then she asked me, "Where do you live?"

I wondered why she wouldn't remember that, but I had moved about five years before. So, after a brief pause and deep thoughts, I said "The Redmond house, you remember, the one with all the horses."

My concern really began with her next comment. She said, "Oh, I think my daughter lives in Redmond; she works in Seattle, but lives in Redmond, drives all that way to work…she really works a lot of long hours… sometimes she doesn't call me until long after dark when she's driving home and I've already cleaned up the dinner dishes…"

Pause — more deep thoughts.

I sat straight up, looked at her square in the face and said, "Mom, I am your daughter."

She just laughed and said, "Oh, I guess you are!"

I tried to dismiss this because I had changed into my bathing suit, and I thought just maybe there was a possibility she could have been confused because she wasn't looking at my face. All the while I was thinking, *my voice was the same and I was her daughter, how could she not know it is me? Her eyesight was fine, her hearing was fine; how could she possibly think I was someone else driving the car or sitting next to her at the pool?*

We continued to enjoy our poolside chat, had a few

snacks and after a little while, we left the pool and ventured out to see the sights. At a local Saturday Market we hoped to find the best deal on locally crafted turquoise and silver jewelry. Something Mom and I shared over the years was the love of shopping and finding a great bargain. I bought a beautiful amethyst necklace and Mom came very close to buying some earrings, but decided to wait and see if she found something else 'down the road.'

Mom was getting tired and hungry. She became fixated on having a baked potato for dinner and brought it up several times. "I really want a nice big baked potato with 'my' butter for dinner"… "Doesn't a baked potato sound good, about now?" We stopped at the store to get potatoes and all the fixings. The 'fixings' were for me; all she wanted was 'her butter.' When we returned to the room, she dozed off while reading her book and I called and checked in with work to tie up any loose ends.

Later, I fixed dinner as she had requested along with the lasagna and salad I had planned the day before, and then there was her baked potato. According to Mom, "The best way to bake a potato is in the oven so that it bakes all the way through and doesn't get those over-baked spots from the microwave." So, potatoes baked in the oven while we sat on the couch with the books we had brought along. When she wondered why dinner was taking so long and I told her the potato needed an hour, she said "I didn't ask you to make a baked potato." She was hungry, getting cranky and now she didn't want the potato after all. I rationalized. It had been before her nap that she had insisted on having one, so maybe she forgot and now I was in my own state of confusion, trying to unravel hers. I decided a joke would be best. As I was thinking, she asked, "Where did that other girl go?"

"I don't know, Mom. I wish she was here; she could have made our dinner!" We giggled together.

Although I was puzzled by her confusion and even a bit annoyed, I continued to rationalize. The new surroundings, for instance: I had taken her out of her own element and thrown her into an entirely different place. That thought prevailed as I argued with myself: *she traveled extensively, had even lived abroad for a time, and was as confident taking the tube in London or sailing on a boat in the Marmara Sea as stepping into her own bathtub.*

The rest of the trip continued to be a learning experience for me as Mom's confusion continued. We lovingly joked around about what 'that other girl' was up to now. I entertained a lot of deep thoughts, reflecting back on phone conversations and other random odd occurrences prior to this trip. The whole family, I felt, had missed many of the early signs. I called home to check in and mentioned that Grandma was a lot more confused than I had thought.

Then came the inadvertent book exchange. We had both brought books to read on the plane and we often relaxed with them, side by side, at the condo. In between times, we left the books on the coffee table. One day, while I was in the kitchen, she picked up my book and started reading it from where I had left my bookmark. When I noticed and asked her why she was reading my book, she tried to convince me it was hers, that she had been reading it all along. Now I thought, *it is one thing to think something is yours because it looks the same, but it's a totally different story to think that you were already reading something you weren't!* I had to go look at the other book to see if maybe I hadn't noticed that we were reading the same book, same author, or something that would explain this confusion. Nope, no similarity at all. "Mom, what makes you think that is your book?" I held up her book. "This one is the one you were reading."

Now I was a little scared, because up to this moment, some of her confusion I had dismissed or rationalized by location, fatigue etc. Since my mother read consistently all throughout my life, I could not comprehend this. I have dyslexia and am a very slow reader and occasionally, when pressed with a homework deadline, Mom would read out loud to help me. Her reading comprehension was admirable as well as her ability to recite content on demand in order to critique my homework assignments. With all these memories ever present in my mind, I could not understand why she didn't stop reading what she couldn't understand, starting in the middle of an unfamiliar book. But, here she was, insisting it was her book and didn't appear to be concerned at all that she didn't know the characters or the storyline.

While I sat there battling with this in my own head, apparently I still wore a puzzled look. She looked at me, really looked at me and said, "What are you looking at me with that face for?"

It was a phrase from my childhood, one I asked as a child once upon a time. As we laughed together, I asked again, "What makes you think that is your book?" Her response wasn't convincing, that she just thought she brought two books, which traditionally was not uncommon for her as she read so fast; she would start a new book right after she finished the last one. But she tried to convince me that it was her book and wouldn't give it back to me. Some stubbornness was naturally ingrained in Mom, but this time she was more insistent and argumentative. I gave up and now, I was the one in a state of confusion. My mother, the avid reader, was gone.

The bottom line became apparent. Her confusion was going to become our journey together, whether I was prepared for it or not.

On the day of departure, we planned our morning over breakfast. We had to pack and I reminded her that our checkout time was noon. In her day, she was a frequent flyer and I expected she knew exactly what that meant. We finished breakfast, got dressed; I cleaned up the kitchen, and got her started packing. I threw my own things and suitcase together and rolled it out by the door. It was getting really close to noon and she was still in her room, so I went to check on her. What a shock! Mom had opened her completely packed suitcase, taken her clothes off and was getting back into bed! I tried not to sound cross when I said, "Mom, what are you doing? We need to go check out."

"I am still tired," was her simple reply. I called the front desk, told them I had a little situation and pleaded for a late checkout. *I really just wanted to sit down and cry, as I was now sure this was not just occasional lapses in memory, or confusion. This was serious.* But, since there wasn't any time for my emotions, I took a very deep breath and coaxed her back to fully dressed, got out the door with all the suitcases and we managed to make it to the airport on time.

Odds and Ends

Early on, before our journey began, I started to notice odds and ends like, "Where are we?" I would remind her which street we were on, and as we were driving, she would say things like, "I don't recognize this area" or 'This doesn't look familiar to me." In some cases, it really concerned me because it was her own neighborhood. She and Dad lived in the same house for nearly sixty years, and although there had been some construction, new homes replacing old, not much had really changed. And certainly not significantly enough to appear unfamiliar.

Like many in their elderly years, Mom needed cataract surgery. She tolerated the surgery well and followed the doctors' orders. We had a daytime caregiver for Dad at this time, so her medications and take-home instructions were monitored by the caregiver. We all checked on her, and she seemed to be doing well. A few days following surgery, Mom called both of my brothers and me with the same complaint. With urgency in her tone, she announced that there was something terribly wrong with the anesthetic that they had used. When I asked what was wrong, she explained that the anesthesia had a horrible side effect and had dried out her skin. "What do you mean," I asked.

"Well, now I have all these wrinkles on my face," she wailed. When I asked what made her think it was the anesthesia, she explained, "Well, I certainly didn't have all these wrinkles before the surgery!" She didn't like my sarcastic response about her improved vision so she called both brothers to see what they thought. Then she said, "That is exactly what your sister said; why don't any of you believe me?" For whatever reason, this experience of anesthesia and wrinkles stuck with her and she never changed her story, or got confused about the details, details that only she recalled.

Scam Artists Prey

Another fear that set in is of the unscrupulous people out there who take advantage of the elderly in their vulnerable years. I don't know if this occurrence was memory loss, gullibility, or just an overly trusting nature, but it was unlike either Mom or Dad to not think things through. Criminals and scam artists abound out there, and they prey on the elderly with well-orchestrated determination.

Mom and Dad went grocery shopping one day at their usual local market. Both of them used a cane when walking, moved slowly and therefore routinely parked in one of the handicapped stalls near the main entrance. As they left the store, the store clerk helped load the groceries into the car. Mom got in the driver's seat and they headed for home via the usual back roads route. A truck came up behind them, honking its horn, and its driver flagged them down. One young man ran over to the car and knocked on the driver's window. Mom slowly got out of the car as he bent down and reached behind the driver's side rear tire and came up with grease on his hands. He showed Mom that there was 'brake fluid' leaking from the wheel. He and his friend could fix it for them, but they needed cash up front.

Now, my Dad could fix anything in his day and he knew a car forwards and backwards, but on this particular day he trusted these two young strangers and did not argue when Mom told him about the leaking fluid. Most of the time Dad did not wear his hearing aids; he may not have even understood what was said. They offered to take Mom home to get her checkbook because she shouldn't drive the car this way, then they could take her to the bank and wait for her while she got cash.

Dad waited there in the car, on a side street near the grocery store, while Mom left because she said she would be right back. Mom got into the pickup with the young man and his son. They drove her home to get her checkbook and then to the bank. Eventually, they returned her to Dad and the car, followed them home again, because the car "wasn't safe to drive," and Mom paid them the $1800 cash. Since they now knew where Mom and Dad lived, they promised to come back in the morning with his friend and the parts to repair the brakes. Of course, the Good Samaritans didn't return. When Mom and Dad realized what had happened, they were ashamed and afraid to tell us that they had been flimflammed. Ultimately, they did tell us and a police report was filed. The police said that this occurs on a regular basis and many a time, their families do not ever know.

Another very common solicitation scam cycle that happened was that they were targeted for every charitable fund there is out there, and they kept making donations to anyone who called. No matter how many times we explained why 'you shouldn't do this,' they forgot the risk and the caller was so believable, they kept writing checks.

Scammed Again

Six months after the brake fluid fiasco, they were scammed again, only this time at home. The con artists must have been watching the house, because they knocked on the front door soon after Dad left for his daily walk. He walked with a walker and had a predictable routine, gone a certain amount of time each day. This time, the team was a man and a young girl. When they came to the door, he told my mom that 'Walt' had asked him to repair the roof over the porch because it was leaking. It wasn't the same young man as the brake scam, but since they knew Mom and Dad by name we think there may have been a relationship network between the con men. The roof wasn't really leaking at that point, but he took a 2 x 4 and pushed it up into the soffit to show Mom how soft the roofing was and made a hole in the shakes to prove it.

Now, Mom trusted that maybe Dad did ask this 'nice man' to repair the roof, so she continued to talk to them. She could just as easily have said "No thanks" but who knows how this might have played out if she didn't cooperate? Once again, she agreed to a ride with 'the man and his daughter.' Mom said the daughter rode in the back seat reading her 'bible' while my mother went into the bank alone. Of course, the 'nice young man' didn't come into the bank with her. Mom said she realized that this was wrong and became nervous when she was in the bank, but since he knew where she lived, she was afraid. She didn't think to tell the bank teller while she was safe inside. He obviously didn't come in with her because of the security cameras, but I doubt Mom realized that. She thought he might come in to see why it was taking her so long. She withdrew $2500 cash for her roof repair and gave it to the man when they got home.

As a concerned family, we each had our own ideas of what she could have or should have done, but later realized that more harm could have come if she had resisted. The roof was never repaired and another report was filed with the police. Mom was clear that she didn't recognize this man as being the same as the brake fluid scam, but the police confirmed that they were most likely linked in some way.

Reeling in the Financial Reins

At that time, my brother, Dennis, started managing their bank accounts for them and basically had to put them on a monitored allowance. If they needed more money, they called and he would transfer it to checking. They no longer had access to their own money beyond grocery shopping and a small amount of cash for meals out. This takeover could have been much more challenging, but due to the scams, they were both appreciative of the help. This turned out to be a wise thing, because it enabled Dennis to control the donations, too. When callers would ask, they would have to say, "I have to ask my son for money," and most callers began to back off. And, if for any reason either of them tried to withdraw a large sum of money from the bank directly, the bank was aware of the situation and had to alert Dennis, since all their funds were now in a trust account and could not be transferred without permission.

We found that if you utilize the rules as commonly followed by the banks, it becomes a check and balance of the system you have put into place. It is a sad time when you have to question your parents' need for money and was certainly a new experience for them. My Dad insisted on keeping a credit card for his mail-order purchases, but Dennis could check the balance online and see where the purchases originated. Since the limit on a credit card can be managed as well as fraudulent activity, this was the stop gap to additional criminal opportunities.

Dad believed that he could take enough herbs to live another 20 years. He believed all the mailings he received promising 'free of back pain forever' and 'cleans your colon for good' offers. It got to the point where he was overmedicating himself with herbs and would not listen to reason from any of us! If it was in writing, it must be true! He became a 'walker walking' dictionary of herb facts. The amazing part of this is that his memory was fine, actually quite sharp for his age. The only symptom he showed was difficulty in finding the right word when he was trying to express himself. He usually wound up swearing and shaking his head, saying "never mind." It took me a while to realize that he was frustrated and not just cranky in his old age. He was six years older than Mom and outside of having a heart condition, healthy in his old age. Eventually he fell and received a serious concussion that caused a subdural hematoma and he had to undergo surgery to relieve the pressure on his brain. During this time, the concussion caused a state of confusion, not unlike the symptoms of Alzheimer's or dementia. Because his normal state of mind was cognitive and in control, when he started asking things like, "Where is the dog?" and "I need to go to work," it alerted us to become concerned.

One day Dad called me, and told me he needed my help. When I asked him what he needed, he said he needed help getting hold of his boss, because he didn't finish a job and needed to get back under this customer's house and he didn't know where the key was. I told him I would stop by on my way home from work and we could talk about it. He said "thank you honey, see you later, bye" and hung up the phone. Dad had been retired since I was fifteen, so I immediately called my brothers and told them what was going on. I, learned that Dad called them also, not making any sense.

When I got to the house, everything appeared normal, Dad was sitting in his favorite chair and Mom was cleaning up the dinner dishes. Mom called me into the kitchen and whispered, "Your dad keeps insisting that he has to go to work, and he gets mad at me when I tell him he doesn't work anymore." When I went into the living room, he told me again that he needed my help finding the phone number for his boss so he could get back into that house. I was thinking, *I don't ever remember*

Dad running electrical wire; he always worked at a desk. So I decided to ask him some more questions and see where this was going.

"Dad, Whose house is it and what did you do under the house?"

"I was hooking up their phone lines," he replied, "and it got too dark and I had to leave, so I need to finish." So I asked him what his boss's name was, and he told me it was Bob and that the phone number was in his black phone book but he couldn't find it. I said I would go look for it, and he thanked me for my help. "Your mother wouldn't help me," he complained. We continued to talk a little bit, in detail about the electrical work he was doing, as I was thinking, *this is kind of cool; he's telling me about a part of his life that was before I can remember as if it was happening right now, but what is going on and why is he so confused?* I called my brothers again, and we decided Dad needed to be checked out so I took him to Emergency and that's how we found out about the concussion.

Dad had a cute 'Little Rascal' scooter and used it to go buzzing down the local bike trail to the market after we took his car keys away. One of the days that he came home on his scooter, he apparently tipped over and hit his head. The neighbor had helped him up and we knew nothing about it other than Mom mentioning that, "Dad drives that thing as crazy as he drove the car." Sometimes you had to put several pieces together to gain the information, as they were used to being independent and unless they 'tattled' on each other, as Mom would put it, we didn't find out. In hindsight, we were creatively kept in the dark most of the time, when they didn't want to get 'caught' or 'scolded.' They were guarding their independence at all costs.

Mom called when Dad began arguing that she lost his dog and what was he going to do because he had to go to work. She said, "There is something strange going on with your father! He thinks I lost Carmel!" When you get these odd phone calls, the reversal happens immediately. They become the child and you the parent. Carmel, their beloved Golden retriever, had been gone for 10 years. We had to ask questions about what had really happened and fortunately were in touch with the neighbors and learned of his Little Rascal incident. The truth was that Dad had raced the mailman to be able to turn into the driveway so he would not have to wait for the mail truck to leave. This race was so typical of his prior driving habits I could not help but chuckle when I heard it. You see, Dad wasn't about to tell us, because he thought we would take away that freedom, too.

Eventually we learned that when he fell, Mom took him to the emergency room and he needed 14 stitches. After the onset of the missing dog confusion, an ER visit, a neurological exam followed by a CT scan, we found out that when he hit his head, he had a serious undiagnosed concussion. As family, you feel that you somehow should have known, and feel responsible. It made us feel lost and out of touch, but we also recognized that they were a difficult pair to manage. You don't want to have every conversation be the 'Grand Inquisition', as Mom put it, but yet, somehow we needed to know when they were at risk. This is where the hired aides became an invaluable resource. The aides would 'tattle' even knowing they were going to hear about it directly from their two charges. Theirs was tough love in action. The circles of newfound truths led to many conversations and family conferences.

My actions today would be to start the communication between siblings earlier on with a method of checks and balances regarding the parents' daily lives in general. As with any family, we all had our own schedules, families, careers and activities, but if we had synchronized our phone calls or visits earlier on, we might have had influence over the progression. I suppose that is my own guilt talking, asking

41

questions such as: Could Mom have started medication sooner? Had we missed a head trauma like Dad's with Mom? All families have concerns and no matter if there wasn't anything that could have been done to change it, we each have a tendency to search for a 'cause' or a point at which we could have changed destiny.

Don't misunderstand me; from where I am now, I don't think we could have changed the outcome, only some of the hiccups in the journey. One can only hope that understanding our journey will help alert you to some hiccups that will occur in your own.

Dad's Surgery

Following Dad's surgery, 24 hour care was essential while his brain healed. He transitioned from the hospital through the rehabilitation center and then on to a private care Home. Dad's care progressed while still in a mild state of confusion, but it was common following this type of surgery. As he expressed more frustration and was determined to go home, it became apparent that he was healing and becoming more himself again. Mom continued to check in on him daily during the six weeks he was in 'the Home' and her own confusion became a minor concern for family while Dad's care took the front seat. During this time, while witnessing Dad's care, Mom expressed her personal preferences regarding her own future. She made it quite clear that she didn't want to be "stuck in some Home, somewhere, with strangers."

Car Keys and When to Stop Driving

My dad was the one who taught us all how to drive. He was as competitive behind the wheel of a car as he was racing his sailboat. A skipper that 'tacked on a dime' and used a stopwatch to time the efficiency of his crew, he was skilled with quick responses. To him, driving was like a game, or even a race. He navigated the road with skilled aggression and wit, complaining when the traffic lights were not synchronized correctly and monitoring his speed to 'check' them. He explained many times how they were supposed to be timed so that you didn't have to stop, and surely not at every signal! So, you can imagine that the man that was in his mind, the 'best driver on the road,' was not an easy takeover. However, we eventually took Dad's car keys away long before Mom's. It was helpful that Mom still drove and didn't like him driving her car. I'm sure it wasn't pleasant for her, but she was fearful for her life with him behind the wheel, so it wasn't a hard sell to get her to drive.

At first, Dad started coming home with parking lot dings in his car, then got into an accident where he made a left turn and did not judge the speed of the oncoming car correctly. Perhaps he just flat out did not see the other car. We never did understand completely what happened, since he still protected his right to drive with less and less information. He thought his reactions and wit were above normal, but in reality, he had slowed in everything he did. Once he had his accident, the car insurance questioned his ability and vision, etc. When his next birthday came around and it was time to renew his driver's license, the insurance required him to retake the written and driving tests. We thought we were out of the woods and our concerns would be resolved without conflict. Well, so much for that idea! Dad managed to pass both tests with flying colors! My brothers complained to the Department of Transportation and learned that because of the strong senior lobbyists protecting their personal rights, family could not influence the licensing process without medical proof of incompetence.

Dad complained that he was having trouble reading, even with his glasses, so Mom made an appointment and took him to the eye doctor. He did have cataracts impairing his vision. His stubborn nature kicked in and he refused to have the surgery no matter how much we tried to convince him otherwise. Dad's cataracts were unfortunate but a helpful side effect used to eventually confiscate his car keys. "Dad's on driving restriction" struck us as funny after all these years, but Dad did not see the humor in it at all.

Did You Take Your Pills?

Medications became another issue. Neither of them could recall if they had taken their pill with breakfast or not, and we don't know how often they either did not, or exceeded their daily dose. When we asked, they would come back with, "of course I did, and don't you think I know how to take care of myself?" I'd think, *'well, actually, no Dad, I don't'*, but that is a tough conversation to have. Dennis also started managing the refilling of prescriptions, keeping track and managing the daily meds with the help of the in home aides we hired. The weekly, three – four compartment boxes of daily doses worked great. Times for pills with meals and at bedtime seemed to fit most of the prescribed doses. As time went on, we became more involved in attending their doctors' appointments with them to make sure that the instructions were followed.

Listen & Ask

I wish I had thought to do a few things while Mom had more clear moments than confused moments. You really don't know how quickly dementia can progress and I took time for granted. I can look back now and see that I was in my own state of denial, too. I have questions about family history, favorite purchases, and even silly things like recipes and stories. There were a lot of stories she told over the years that I just don't remember clearly - who moved where and when, what my great grandfather on my father's side did for a living, etc. Whatever happened to Grandpa's paintings? My grandfather on my mother's side was an artist in addition to being a barber, but I never had the opportunity to see his artwork. I wish I had Mom write names on the back of family photos. There are slews of old family pictures from our heritage, but I can't tell Aunt Dora from Auntie Lucille. Whatever you think you or your children may want to know and have never taken the time to ask, don't put it off any longer. If it's not already too late, do it now! If you don't have time to write it all down, record a few conversations and you can reflect on it later when you have the time. A good time to ask questions is while driving together in the car. I found that isolated time very productive, but of course couldn't write anything down while driving; I wish I had thought to record it.

Dad would mention on occasion that he didn't think Mom was "right in the head." It was hard to be there at the right moment to see what he meant, and he couldn't always clearly describe the situations, or recall all the details. Although older than Mom, he still managed to consistently maintain a good memory. It is much easier to look back in that rearview mirror of life and see where I have been, than it is to see what is down the road ahead. The only advice I can pass on at this point is to confront the issue, no matter how difficult it is, even when you are dealing with your parents. They may not like it, but 'helping' is a good way to spend time and analyze what is really going on. My brothers would show up to look at a leak in the basement, or inspect something on the property that they thought might need a repair. With an older home, those incidents were as numerous as you can imagine. Dad was still convinced he could climb up a ladder and fix a leaky gutter, so they had to be creative and just do it. They would let him 'help' or more accurately, 'supervise' and direct them. Dad had been actively teaching us all our lives, so that part had not changed much.

Those Nice Firemen Stopped By Again

A security system was installed early on; Mom and Dad just had to remember to use it if and when the time arose. There were two keypads, one upstairs by the front door and the other in the downstairs hallway. The keypads had pre-programmed buttons for Fire, Medical and Police. Dennis had written in large letters and taped them next to each corresponding button so that they were easier to see and understand than the small symbols typically used. One night there was a windstorm and the power went out after Mom and Dad went to bed. I am not sure what the sequence of events was, but it was at a time when they had daytime only caregivers, so they were home alone through the night without power. They now had separate bedrooms, primarily because Mom said "your dad snores so loud he could wake the dead."

Apparently, Mom got up first, a little disoriented in the darkness, and fell while trying to find her way down the short hallway to the bathroom. She must have called for Dad and when he got up and tried to get to her, he either tripped over her or somehow fell, too. As they both lay on the floor in the dark, they could not see or figure out where they were and Mom's confusion made it even more difficult. Due to their age, getting up off the floor had its own challenges. Somehow, Dad got his bearings and crawled to the wall where the Alarm Keypad was; its battery backup kept the buttons lit and he was able to push the 911 medical emergency button. The response team called immediately, but he couldn't answer because he could not find the phone in the dark.

As Mom described the event, 'the nice firemen' came to the door, and Dad crawled up the stairs to let them in. After they thoroughly checked both of them over, illuminated by their flashlights, they helped Mom and Dad safely back to bed. When they called Dennis, the emergency contact, they gave him the update and suggested that his parents really should not be living alone. After this incident, care was arranged and one of the caregivers stayed at the house overnight, providing us with some peace of mind.

The little room that Mom called the den was adjusted to accommodate a small bed and a dresser, and worked well for overnight caregivers. Mom clearly expressed, "I don't want strangers in my house! I will have to watch every move they make and I just don't have the time to babysit and chitchat."

My parents were blessed to have good team of nurturing and loving staff as their caregivers. Mom thought they were there to help her take care of Dad. Dad thought they were there to keep Mom from nagging him, keep her entertained and cook. Either way, it worked. I wish I could say everything was happy-go-lucky and without any hiccups, but that wouldn't be how life goes, now would it?

Dad had a bit of a temper and had spoken his mind all my life. So when Claudette called and said Dad had yelled at her and called her a stupid broad, I wasn't surprised. I apologized and asked her what had happened. When Dad tried to explain how to check and see why the phone next to his chair wasn't working, she didn't follow his directions exactly the way he wanted. Since he had been an engineer for the phone company, in his mind his way was the right way to do it. Claudette found that out the hard way when she picked up the other phone to see if all the phones were out rather than move the table next to Dad's chair and unplug his phone and take it to another jack to see if it worked there as Dad had instructed. The bottom line was, none of the phones worked because the phone service was out. But, in Dad's mind, he was her boss and she didn't listen!

I promised to come by on my way home from work and make my dad apologize and explain to him why he can't call her a stupid broad even if he believed he was right. Most of the time Dad was agreeable and appreciative of the home cooked meals and companionship. He would not let the aides help him shower, however, and used that as an excuse not to shower at all. Telling him to do anything that he had made up his mind not to do was always a challenge. One day I threatened to roll his wheelchair into the back of my truck and drive him through the car wash if he didn't take a shower. And with that, I had to point out that he was beginning to smell like the compost bin. I made him laugh and he agreed that one of the male aides could help him shower.

Why was he being so stubborn? Then it occurred to me, oh so sadly, that this was one more form of independence being taken away from Dad. A man who could always care for himself and take care of others, was unable to shower without help.

Mom did not like having strangers in her house, period. The aides that could cook to her standards were gradually allowed to cook. She became accustomed to having help in the form of cleaning and shopping and was grateful for it. But while they were in her house she wore herself out, because she still felt they couldn't be trusted and therefore followed them around, watching every task they did.

As a result of her constant fears that they would "steal something right from under my nose," she started hiding things. When she couldn't find them again, she would call me and rant and rave about things that were missing. I can't tell you how many times I heard the "I told you this wasn't a good idea, I don't trust them for a minute!" lecture. Mom was a stubborn woman and once she got something stuck in her head, it was nearly impossible to bring her around, even with early-onset dementia. Gradually the caregivers succeeded in gaining the trust and respect of both our parents, which made life easier for all of us.

Mom and Dad were always very close with their neighbors. One particular neighbor was an elderly woman who lived alone, and became accustomed to Mom bringing her dinner daily. Mom said she "had to cook anyway, so it wasn't a bother at all." Mom would routinely dish up three plates of food and walk over next door, knock and take dinner to Alice.

Later, after dinner, Alice would call Mom and say "thank you, it was very delicious," and she always complimented Mom's cooking. Then, the next morning Dad would go over with the morning paper, visit and pick up the dinner plate from the night before. This neighborly habit went on for many years. When the aides started cooking, Mom would ask them to make enough for Alice and take it over to her. I had to explain that on occasion, Mom forgot that Alice had died. I remember the morning when Dad went to take Alice her paper, and didn't find her downstairs. He went upstairs to find her still in bed. After he made the appropriate phone calls, he came home and told Mom that Alice had died in her sleep. After they shared their grief with each other, Mom said "I hope it wasn't my dinner!"

Looking For Care

On their fixed income, they really could not afford to continue twenty four hour care, or supervision, as I called it. Although they had managed for quite some time with in home, dawn to dusk care, it was apparent now that it was time to consider alternative care. There was a very nice assisted living facility close to their familiar neighborhood, and we placed them on a waiting list. The big question remained: how were we going to convince them to move? They had lived in one house for nearly sixty years and had almost literally grown roots. Well, we managed to come up with some pretty good reasons about home repairs, painting etc. and convinced them that they could have two separate small apartments side by side and would still eat together and participate in the activities in the facility.

Don't think that this was a quick or easy transition. Like any change, when it came to the new location, they had mixed feelings. Dad adjusted much quicker than Mom and just loved it. It was right next to Northgate shopping mall and he had a newfound freedom, since he had not been driving for some time. He still had his Little Rascal scooter and could ride it down the elevator, up a half a block to the corner traffic light, cross the street and be at the mall. He buzzed around to all the shops, filled up his basket and ran his 'errands' just like the good old days.

Mom, on the other hand, was obstinate and complained about everything. She missed her house, she didn't like the food, she couldn't sleep there in 'that bed', regardless of the fact that it was the same bed, with the same linens, just in a different location. Mom always prepared the meals, and had expressed her feelings that she was *tired of cooking* and this was completely understandable after 60 some years of marriage and we respected how she felt. We really thought that having someone else fix their meals would be a big plus. Not so much. She actually went on an eating strike. She refused to eat their food and lost 10 pounds while they lived there. Talk about stubborn. There was nothing wrong with the food; we ate there with them and it was well- presented, tasty and balanced, nutritious meals. But she would look at the menu posted in the elevator and start complaining before she ever got to the dining room. Her mind was made up and there was no changing it. "Your dad needs to be here, not ME!"

Mom still had her car and they could leave and go out to dinner or shopping whenever they needed, but that still was not enough freedom to satisfy her.

"When is the work at the house going to be done," Dad asked. "Your mother is driving me nuts; she does not like it here!" So, that plan turned out to be a family experience in semi-dependent living for the very independent adults in our life. Between Mom's eating strike and Dad's frustration with her, we cried 'Uncle', arranged for 24 hour care and they happily moved back home.

Within a year of our Phoenix excursion, Dad was diagnosed with pancreatic cancer and died soon after his diagnosis. It all happened too quickly for all of us, but especially for Mom. The day we brought Dad home from the hospital under the supervision of Hospice, we had a family gathering at the house. Dad loved having his family around him. In a sense, it was as reassuring for him as it was us.

We set up the hospital bed by his favorite window with a view, which allowed him to be at home with family as he wished. I was hobbling around on crutches healing a broken leg. Once at the house, I stayed and helped care for Dad. We set up the hospice-provided pharmacy in the kitchen with gloves, moisturizing sponges, syringes, morphine, and the dosage instructions. Mom seemed to understand every step, watched our every move. I slept on the couch, she in her bed and others went home at night and returned in the morning. Following the hospice guidelines, we watched for the end of life signs. As prescribed, I set a timer on my phone for morphine dosages every two hours.

The now-familiar timer rang on this windy Saturday morning. I hobbled to the kitchen where Dennis and Mom were cleaning up the dishes. When I returned with the morphine syringe, Dad had stopped breathing. The guidebook said that he might go for long periods between breaths as he neared the end. As I watched his chest for movement, I called out, "I think it's time" to Dennis and Mom. We three stood at his side, holding his hands, telling him he was free to go see his sister, his mother, his father and his best friend who fell overboard in heavy winds on Dad's sailboat.

Dennis held Mom in his arms and guided her up the steps to her bedroom to rest while we waited for the coroner. Two young gentlemen dressed in suits arrived, politely introduced themselves, expressed their condolences and went to work. As they quietly and respectfully took care of Dad, Dennis and I stood watching the cloud-covered sky in silence. Mom joined us outside to say goodbye. We three watched as the black covered bag laid out on the gurney quietly slid into the long black hearse. With a handful of Kleenex bunched in her hand, Mom waved goodbye as the hearse drove away and stood there in the middle of the street while it disappeared down the lane.

Dad passed within two days of the gathering, but in Mom's memory, "Dad died at the party." She could not be convinced otherwise. I believed that she just blocked out the two long and sad days while he was medicated and sleeping and passed quietly with us by his side. Mom's confusion seemed to worsen rapidly after Dad died. While at the hospital and at Dad's deathbed all through his last days, she seemed at peace and relieved that he did not suffer. Her confusion became more apparent to us as we spent extra time with her, comforting her through her grief and making sure she could live alone for a little while. While we each shared our concerns, she did not seem in any immediate danger.

As I have witnessed all of these experiences over time and can look back from a distance, I came to the conclusion that dementia helps us to avoid and even escape uncomfortable memories. In most cases this is possibly a blessing.

Mom did not want to leave her home, actually refused to do so, so we continued with the part-time in home care we had previously arranged. She started to exhibit much more assertive behavior than we had seen before. She became argumentative and was dead set that she was right, even in her state of confusion. She did fine with the part time in-home arrangements for a while, until she started leaving the teakettle to boil dry or forgetting she had turned the oven on.

Once, I arrived after work and an odd odor assailed my nostrils when I opened the front door. Yes, the tea kettle had burned dry and the metal was so hot it glowed red. Immediately, safety measures were put in place, monitored smoke detectors and a personal call for help alert device that she wore around her neck. She could push a button if she fell or needed help and could communicate with an emergency response center via speakerphone. It provided some comfort knowing that if she did need help, she could get it. There were also caring neighbors that would check on her and help us if we could not reach her by phone.

Don't Even Think About Taking My Car Keys!

The time came when we realized that it just wasn't safe for Mom to drive any longer. I never really had thought about how hard it would be to take anyone's independence away. Taking the keys was not as simple as it sounded. We tried to tell her we were worried and we didn't want her driving, but that went absolutely nowhere because, "I am fine; I don't know what you are all worried about, I have been driving for many years longer than any of you are old!!" This wasn't just someone, this was our mother. Besides our obvious fear that she'd have an accident, we worried that she would get lost. She had begun to make comments like, "What's the name of the long street up the hill from my house?" not knowing what street she was on and "things just look different."

Over time, it became even more apparent that Mom shouldn't be driving any longer. Dennis tried to tell her and she would hear nothing of it. "You are not telling me what I can and cannot do; I am still your mother!"

The inevitable happened. Dennis got a call from the

caregiver one morning at 8 a.m. "Corrine is leaving for her hair appointment and it isn't until 10 a.m.," she said. He asked why, since it only took 10 minutes to get there? She explained that Mom thought that she had to leave earlier because we had moved her house.

By day's end, we had all had variations of this same conversation with her. She continued to insist that she lived in the same house and yes, everything was the same but we had moved it and now it took her much longer to get to the hairdresser. I asked questions like, "Does John still live next door? Is the trail still across the street?" She answered all those questions correctly, but insisted that we had moved the house. We came to believe she must have had that I am lost feeling any time she left the neighborhood. Who knew which way she was planning to drive, that could lead to a ten minute drive taking two hours? Of course, we arranged for a ride to her appointments from then on.

As she grew more and more confused, it was in her best interest that we lost her car keys. She looked for days and Dennis arranged to have her ride with a neighbor to the store. Then she found her second set of keys and began driving again. But she would say, "I went to the store and…" And then when you caught her in the midst of her own story, she would say, "Don't tell your brother, he thinks I shouldn't drive any longer." She thought we were still separate and not teaming up against her, but by now we were comparing notes and communicating often.

Then, Dennis got creative. He disconnected the distributor and told her that there was something wrong with the car and it wouldn't start. She kept calling and nagging each of us to get the car fixed. Then she outfoxed us! She called AAA and had someone come look at it. They reconnected the distributor and once again, she was driving. We were grateful that she didn't understand that the car problem was due to our undermining mechanical methodology.

I commend your efforts and wish you luck while thoughtfully diminishing your loved one's independence, 'one damn thing after another,' as Dad had scolded. If they are cooperative and agreeable, consider your plan a great success. If they are uncooperative, try to carry out the plan with a grace that allows them to still feel in control of the choices. Be as understanding as possible. Control is slowly being delegated to you, a foreign concept to a parent.

Brother Rick's bright idea was to buy Mom's car from her for a good price. We all thought that by selling it to family, she could still ride in it. He made the effort to pick her up in it for family gatherings, thinking she might appreciate it, but instead she scolded him for stealing her car.

I eventually heard many of the stories she told to her friends. In her confused state, believing that we were "out to get her," she apparently had convinced friends that her family was neglecting her and being unkind to her. While we were in the throes of making choices about safety and searching for quality care, we had not considered having to defend those decisions to others. I felt hurt that Mom had painted the picture shaded with unkind intentions. In reflection, I can imagine that she was simply looking for sympathy from sources that listened and gave her the responses she needed to hear as the unwelcomed changes ensued.

We made arrangements with a neighbor to invite Mom to go grocery shopping or to call and check to see if she needed anything. Rick's wife, BJ, also called on a regular basis to get a grocery list and delivered easy and healthy options to cook. Since Mom was on her own much of the time for dinner, she would choose the easiest options and was therefore eating much less healthy food. I couldn't say that I blamed her, after all the years she cooked for us. I'm all for the easy menu, but BJ dropped by one day with groceries and found Mom in the kitchen eating Cool Whip from the plastic tub she had just pulled from the freezer. Mom was always health conscious and this posed a multifaceted concern. Did she think it was ice cream or did she just like the sweet taste?

Pets

Mom always had dogs, and now that she was alone, she must have felt a companion would help. She had asked and we had talked about it, but recognized that she was having enough difficulty managing a cane and the stairs in the house without the responsibility of a dog. We had to tell her we were sorry, but we did not think it was a good idea. One of her well-meaning friends thought it would be a great idea to give Mom a sweet dog from the animal rescue shelter, and didn't consult the family. This turned out to be a bad idea. It was good in the sense that Sadie proved to be a loving companion, but Mom didn't remember if she had let the dog out or not, fed the dog or not and it soon became the added responsibility of the caregiver. Also, there was construction next door and the fence was not secure, so she had to take the dog out on a leash. I was constantly worried that Mom would get the leash tangled up in her cane and fall.

Although Sadie was a dear companion, the poor dog was overweight because Mom continually fed her table scraps. I reminded her often that it wasn't healthy for Sadie. The dog would beg, and Mom would say, "Aw, she is so cute, just look at her," and the don't-feed-her-people-food rule went out the door.

A companion animal is a great idea, with the right arrangements. A cat and a litter box is probably a better idea than an 85 lb. Labrador Retriever that needs a bathroom escort, on a leash, several times a day.

Laughter Still Lives Here

Over time, the aides became part of our family. On occasion, I called ahead and invited Mom out to lunch or dinner and she and her caregiver *du jour* would meet me at a restaurant. One day we met for lunch and there were six ladies in all. We enjoyed a nice family style lunch as a group, at a cozy Italian restaurant. When the check came we were trying to split the bill and calculate the tip. As the check was circulating around the table with discussions of who ate what and who owed what, Mom interrupted, pulled her emergency call necklace from around her neck, waved it in the air and asked, "Do you want me to call for help?"

As we were all laughing with her, I wondered *how does she manage to still have her quick wit amidst all of the confusion? And then I couldn't help but wonder if she understood that the emergency necklace only worked at home where the monitor base was?* It was a good time, a good day and that story has been treasured by all who were blessed to go to lunch with Mom that day. When BJ came by, she would often bring a lady she was helping care for along for the outing. Her name was Mary Jean and she was losing her eyesight and therefore a little timid in new places. When Mom greeted Mary Jean, she would say, "Well if it isn't Esmeralda Sue Hickenlooper!" In response to this greeting, Mary Jean would giggle and feel immediately at ease. Mary Jean and Mom were quite a team as they were both forgetful and the ensuing conversations were rather comical. The entertainment reoccurred on a semi-weekly basis for six plus months until Mary Jean needed full time professional care. Long afterward, Mom would mention them and ask BJ, "Where is that Esmeralda Sue Hickenlooper?"

Budget Decisions: Searching For Quality Care

As time went on, the care necessary for Mom to live at home became too expensive because she needed 24 hour supervision. My brothers and I searched all the local options and discovered a wide variety of care. Although there was a long list to choose from, it takes time to do all the necessary research. It was a process of first calling doctors and friends for referrals, then calling the list to see if they had openings and then making a list of which ones to check out.

Our choices were: In- home care, Assisted Living, Memory Care, Transitional Care, Private Home care and Traditional Nursing Home care.

In-home care: Allows the patient to continue to live at home, with help providing various tasks as needed. Staff available part time to full time and 24 hour care options available. If arranged through a service, billed by the hour. Standard minimum hours per week are 18 hrs. This allows the service to schedule the same caregivers familiar with the patient as much as possible. This is the type of care Mom and Dad used while living in their own home. Rates vary geographically, in Seattle rates started at $18 hr. The aides received $12 hr. wage. The advantage of staffing through a service is that they cover the shift with an alternate, allowing time off for the aides as necessary.

Hiring individuals directly is also a viable option. It puts you in control of who is hired and you manage the care via your own staff of caregivers. The downside is managing it as a business, with employee wages, tax liabilities and time off coverage etc. This option can work well if you have the flexibility in your own life to step in as caregiver as needed.

Assisted Living: Provides semi-independent living within a safe community with a variety of care options based on the individual needs of the patient. Customary small apartment units with a kitchenette and private bathroom. Studio and one or two bedroom apartments for couples, or options to share a bathroom and kitchenette with a private bedroom for each resident. Private phones for each resident and meals and activities are available and optional. The maximum additional care options are bath aides, scheduled checking in on resident. The care coordinator is the point of contact for care plan coordination and special arrangements. This situation is valuable allowing safety in independent living, but usually doesn't offer 24-hr patient monitoring as an option.

Memory Care: is a community of residents with similar symptoms. Alzheimer's and Dementia run side by side, affecting patients' short term memory. These facilities provide care from staff trained specifically in dealing with these unique symptoms. Care can be offered in a variety of living situations and can also provide a support network for the patients' families.

Transitional Rehabilitative Care: Nursing home structure, short term rehabilitative care is available after discharge from a hospital. Less expensive than hospital care.

Private Home care: as an independent small business, private homes can be a personalized experience. The layout of the homes vary as much as any residential home, however provide semi-independent living. Private bedroom, shared bath. Meals served as a group or in patient's private room.

Traditional Nursing Home Care: Is a full care facility offering patient management under doctor's orders similar to a hospital setting. Group activities and community dining provides social interaction for residents interested in participating. There are a variety of care options within a nursing home as the patient's needs change. Anything from hair appointments to physical therapy and doctor's appointments can all be managed without leaving the Home.

Costs associated with each of these options vary considerably. Payment options are: Medicare, Private insurance coverage and Private pay.

It is best to reach out to Alzheimer's Organization's local chapter for your community to request a list of quality care options that will fit the patient's situation.

The best care available usually has the longest waiting list but, due to the nature of the business, openings do become available. Plan ahead and be patient. Touring the various Homes is an essential part of the process of finding quality care. For some Homes, we just stopped by to see what our first impression was. This provided a real everyday picture of the conditions and care. It was an experience I will never forget! In some situations, the smell was the biggest turnoff. I understand that bodily elimination is a natural part of what is managed and that timing could have played a part in our visits, however, it had a memorable impact. When we came upon a Home that smelled fresh as you walked through the door, it was reassuring that those bodily functions were well managed.

Cleanliness, atmosphere, safety, staffing and staff turnover were at the top of our list. The availability of medical care, procedures for communication between staff and family and the pricing structure were next on the list. After we narrowed down the list, we took the leap and started introducing the idea to Mom. Reluctantly, she toured and gave her honest opinions. We filtered through her stubbornness and whittled down the list by watching how she interacted with the staff. After weeks of searching, we found a nice facility that specialized in memory care. This is a wonderful plan if the opportunity is available in your area. It was classified as assisted living and they had several small apartment style options. As we toured the Home and talked about what Mom liked and didn't like, I will let you guess which list was longer.

The entrance was much like a hotel style lobby with the dining room to the left. As you entered through the double doors, the fragrance of home baked cookies lured you to the dining counter. The dining tables were covered with white linen tablecloths and fresh flowers were on each table. I noticed that they used real glass and silverware as opposed to another we toured that had the feel of an industrial cafeteria. We left the assisted living place with a set of plans of the many room designs to choose from. After some lengthy discussions and budget review, we all agreed on the unit Mom chose. It was a small apartment with a sizable bath and cozy bedroom/ living area and she could have her own furniture there which made her feel comfortable. Yes, she resisted every step of the way. She refused to eat their food, complained about the staff and it took quite a while to get her bearings. We just kept visiting and working with the staff to get her used to her new Home. It took her a couple of months to settle in and get acquainted.

Where Did My Mommy Go?

I had a big party for my 50th Birthday and it was important to me to involve Mom as much as possible in the planning. After all, she had been a part of every birthday party that I could recall. But, it was soon evident that her state of mind couldn't track a progression of event planning any longer. This was tough for me to accept, though as the illness progresses you will witness every painful step of the journey in living color. Our individual and personal memorable moments of the past can be jolted into a new reality when something that was once simple and routine has suddenly become unclear in the parent's mind. A mother, always before a take-charge woman, the queen of planning family parties, was now lost in a guest list of names she couldn't remember.

We sat there at the table together with the list in front of us, as she read the names aloud and had no recollection of the person attached to the name. She asked, "Who is this?" as she pointed to one of the names. I looked at her, puzzled that Jan, my lifelong friend since kindergarten did not remain in her heart and mind. To Mom, it was just a list of strangers. Each day was becoming a new experience for both of us. This seemed like such a small thing, but it was another part of my mom that I was really going to miss.

She was more like her old self when it got closer to the party date, and was able to come and enjoy herself. I had loads of food and a live band. Mom danced with family and friends and was the life of the party, just like old times. She always loved music and dancing and if she was confused, it went unnoticed and I believe she actually remembered it was my birthday!

The Sprinklers Are Moving Around on the Ceiling

Once Mom was situated in her new mini apartment, everything seemed to be going smoothly. We all checked in regularly and gave her lots of attention. Overall, I was very pleased with the care and this time she seemed to be eating without any indication of or a reenactment of the hunger strike. Thank God, she forgot that trick! Dennis installed a phone in her room and we posted a list of all of our phone numbers so she could always reach us if needed. She called randomly just to chat, but she went through a period of calling after she went to bed and she seemed to be afraid. There was her overall confusion of not remembering where she was and then a new concern that lasted for a couple of weeks. She would call and say, 'They are doing it again!"

"What is doing it again, Mom?"

"There are these white round things on my ceiling and the things that the water comes out of and they move every night." I did not understand what she meant, but tried to reassure her that everything was fine and said we could talk about it in the morning. She apparently called both Dennis and Rick after we hung up and they each had the same conversation. Later, Dennis figured out she was referring to the smoke detectors and sprinkler heads.

She had a night light next to the bed so we thought perhaps the 'moving things' were shadows. At least, we tried to rationalize what was apparently a hallucination. This behavior stopped, and after a few conversations with the staff at the Home and Mom's doctor, it was thought that maybe she was having a reaction to a new medication intended to help her sleep at night. I learned that there are many factors involved with dementia, and at times symptoms were a side effect to medication, not to be confused with a normal state of confusion.

Wow! There I was, translating normal confusion from medicated confusion and all the while becoming more confused myself.

All this time, I had trouble within my own mind, accepting that we had put Mom in a Home, like she did not want to do to her own mother. I continued to feel a sense of guilt for not being able to care for her myself. By the time she needed expensive care, I had purchased her house and she had the funds in reserve to be self-sufficient for a while. However, we could not rule out the possibility of needing financial assistance over her life expectancy. Since Grandma had lived until she was 102 and Mom was currently quite physically healthy, her duration of need for care was unknown. At one point, I talked to Dennis and Rick about the possibility of finishing the basement that Dad had never completely finished. I thought if we could create a little cozy apartment in the 500 square feet, then I could care for her on evenings and weekends. I had updated a bathroom with a wheelchair accessible shower but was still a long way from finishing the rest of the project. Nor could I afford to fund the improvements at that time.

Then there was the reality of what it means to have the responsibility of a loved one under your roof, caring for all their needs. Mom and Dad had cared for both of my father's parents when the time came, as well as Gram Gram, my maternal grandmother. There wasn't any question for them as to any imposition, they just did it. Mom was working full time when Grandma lived with them. I cannot remember how long that was, but I believe it was at least a couple of years. Faced with this choice myself, I struggled with the responsibility and our relationship. Once you have left home and been on your own, having your mother stay for a sleepover or going on vacation was an entirely different journey than providing full care. Still, knowing that I honestly don't think I would have had the patience,

I felt bad for not at least giving it a shot.

It doesn't do me any good to beat myself up because I didn't attempt to care for Mom at home. It is important to know what you are capable of and what you are not. In this case, I can say it, but I still have trouble freeing myself from the twinges of unresolved guilt.

Lynne's Birthday Party

My cousin Lynne was having her 70th birthday party and I knew that Mom would want to be there. I coordinated the arrangements with the Home to have her all dressed and ready, and I would pick her up, allowing plenty of time for the drive. When I arrived, Mom apparently had told the staff at the Home that I was getting married. So when they congratulated me I didn't understand why so I said, "Oh it's not my birthday, it's my cousin Lynne's."

After explaining to the staff that it was definitely not my wedding, we rushed through getting her downstairs and into the car. Mom was seated in the front seat next to me and we headed out for the 45 minute drive. After we pulled out onto the main road, Mom asked me, "How did you know he was the right one?"

I said. "Who?"

"The man."

I asked, "What man?"

"That man you haven't introduced me to yet!"

Ok, this was really getting confusing, what the heck was she talking about? Then it dawned on me.

"Mom, what on earth makes you think I'm getting married; we are going to Lynne's party."

"Oh, that's right." *Good* I thought, *now this is done!*

As I detoured through an espresso stand to order two lattés, "Who did the invitations?"

"Lynne's granddaughter," I answered.

"And what about the flowers?"

I said, as I handed her a mocha latte, "Did you want to get her flowers?"

Just as I took a sip of my coffee, she said, "No, the flowers for your wedding."

Oh, for heaven's sake, I thought, *we're back there again.* I could hardly swallow fast enough to say "Mom, I am not getting married, there is no man and we are going to Lynne's birthday party!" There was nothing but silence from the passenger seat until we were nearly there. Then: "What does Steve think of him?" Steve was my ex-husband and she loved him dearly.

This whole dementia thing is a crock, I thought; *there is nothing wrong with her ability to still annoy the heck out of me.*

I needed to distract her from the topic locked and loaded in her mind. So I asked, "We're almost to Lynne's, do you want to put on some lipstick?"

"I don't have my purse; what did you do with my purse?"

While waiting for the signal to change, I handed her two lipsticks from my purse and said, "Here Mom, I forgot your purse, you can use mine. Choose the one you like best and you can keep it in your pocket." Knowing perfectly well that we took her purse away because she kept leaving it behind, it was easier to bite my tongue than to bring that up again. As I flipped the visor and mirror down so she could see, I noticed a hair under her chin and pulled out my tweezers. "Mom, look at me for a minute, let me get that witch hair from under your chin."

"Ouch! Be careful with that or I'll put your head in the pencil sharpener!"

How does she do that? A phrase she has said for years just flows off her tongue without a hitch but she can't remember what day it is?

At the next stoplight, I started to reach over towards her chin and she grabbed the tweezers out of my hand.

"I can do it myself!"

It was a very long ride, and when we arrived, my brothers came out to the car to help. As we got the wheel chair out of the back and while Dennis and Rick were helping Mom out of the car, BJ asked how it went "I'll explain," I breathed, "but first I need one of Lynne's famous martinis."

After they wheeled Mom into the house and everyone said their hellos, Mom took center stage in a loud voice. "I thought we were going to Faith's wedding!"

I just headed to the counter in search of a martini glass, shrugged my shoulders and said, "Apparently, Mom found the man of my dreams but she can't remember his name."

Honorary 50 Year Members at Church

Mom was a member of the same neighborhood church since it opened. They were having an event during the anniversary service to honor their lifetime members and Mom was invited. My son, Sam, and I decided to take her to be recognized. I asked the Home to please be sure she was up, dressed and finished with her breakfast by 9AM, which would allow just enough time for us to get there in time for the 10AM service.

At the church, Mom was invited to sit in the front pew so that she could stand up when the time of recognition came. She was in her usual state of confusion and the hostess asked if I thought my mother would like to say a few words. I thought about it, and told her that I honestly had no idea what she might say. Since she had been on many a stage, even though this was her church, I didn't know if she would think she had to sing, or perform or could track why she was there. So, I was anxious when the time came.

They did a very nice job recognizing every honorary member. Sam helped her walk up front and while all six of the silver haired honorary members were proudly standing in front, they passed the microphone and asked if there was anything each of them wanted to say. A few people commented, and when Mom's turn came, I was on the edge of my seat.

She took the microphone, cleared her throat and with her customary beautiful smile, graciously thanked everyone for coming. I teared up with pride that she won the audience over and was overcome with relief that she did not in any way embarrass herself. We sang hymns together just like old times except, the new high tech replacement for the hymn book was a full sized screen above the pastor's head, scrolling the words for each verse. But, hymnals were still in the pews and I quickly found the hymn in the book for her. Reading the words on the big screen seemed to confuse her.

Following the service, they had a nice reception in their new congregation hall. They had expanded the building since I was last there. Instead of the old musty church basement, windows surrounded us with a view of the sunlit greenbelt behind the church. I got us each a cup of coffee while the hostess was cutting the cake. Mom didn't want any cake at the reception, so when it was served I only brought one piece back to the table. I sat down and took a bite and then she demanded, "Who took my cake?" I told her she said she didn't want any, and she replied, "I certainly do, too; it is my party, not yours!"

She spoke in her loud mother voice, as she scolded me for not bringing her cake, and others in the congregation hall began to pay attention. While I replayed in my mind asking her if she wanted cake, for my own peace of mind, one of the church elders that had also been recognized knew Mom and came over to see if he could assist. Always a big flirt with the men, Mom immediately brightened up when he offered to get her some cake. "Well thank you for thinking of me," she smiled, "and yes, I would love some cake." I smiled at her youthful bliss and thanked him with a wink.

It was a good day, and one that I didn't want to end. The sun was nearly straight overhead when we left the church, so I headed the car toward the restaurant where Mom's neighbors often had their Sunday brunch. Sure enough, Cory's car was in the parking lot.

Claire's Pantry hadn't changed since I was in Junior High. The odor of freshly baked cinnamon rolls was exactly the same. It assaulted our nostrils the moment we opened the front double door, and it seemed like Mom remembered as she sniffed. I felt at home and was sure Mom did, too, as we approached the hostess.

Why, of course we could go and look for our friends, she smiled as she waved us on. Past the bar and its slight odor of stale cigarettes and beer, we made Mom's grand entrance into the lounge, and there they were, all six of them sitting in their favorite spot by the windows at a corner table. She was in rare form and her audience didn't let her down. "Corrine," Louise shouted. They had been friends since they were pregnant with Cory and me, fifty years ago, and neighbors all that time. "How wonderful to see you out and about again," Louise went on. "Come, sit next to me!" Chuck, Louise's husband, stood up and asked the waitress to pull over another table and chairs as he greeted Mom with a big hug. Cory's younger brother, Eric, and his niece, Jessica, adjusted their chairs to make room for us.

Mom, I realized, had never met Cory's wife, Milari, and I made the introductions. "Cory is married?" Mom was bemused. Without even a 'pleased to meet you,' she said "Well, my dear, what made you want to marry Cory?"

Chuck and Louise had attended Dad's memorial service we had at the house, and I reminded Mom that Cory and Milari were on their honeymoon when Dad died. Cory apologized again how sorry he was that he had not been there for Mom.

"Corrine, you and Walt have always been like a second set of parents for me! He put his arm around her shoulders and squeezed her tight.

I ordered a senior eggs with toast for Mom and eggs Benedict for me, while she entertained Louise's family with stories of Cory dancing on her coffee table as a kid, and of the wild youngster he had been – fast cars in high school and all that went with his teen years. While I was catching up with Milari, Louise ordered Mom a glass of chardonnay, her friend's favorite wine.

Cory told Mom how much he missed Walt's words of wisdom, and told us all tales about Dad. "Walt always seemed to be outside when I drove by and he still waved his arms wildly - yelling at me to 'slow down' just as he did when I was in high school!" Cory occasionally stopped by and visited with my parents when he was in the neighborhood. Milari and Mom discovered that they had both worked at Nordstrom and knew some of the same people.

At least one more glass of wine was ordered and willingly consumed, and I know Mom was a little tipsy when she hugged everyone goodbye. *What the heck*, I thought, *she doesn't get much of a chance to live it up with all her food and beverages controlled at the Home.* This outing had to be good for her; it was just like old times.

Sunday afternoon dinner was still going when we got back, the homey smell of roast pork and gravy permeating the cafeteria's air. Most of Mom's acquaintances were still at tables, many with family who had come to share a meal that day, and all beckoned to her to come and join them. "How was church," was the question most asked.

Corrine Louise Marshall was loud and proud. All ears in the dining room were tuned to her voice. "Very, very nice," she declared. "I loved the music. And they even served my favorite wine."

Phone Calls

Rick always called Mom to tell her when 'the game' was on and what time and channel. This was seasonal, of course - Mariners in the spring and summer, Seahawks in the fall, along with Huskies football or basketball. Mom always enjoyed sports, and Rick shared her joy. The routine began years before when they would call each other before and after games, exchanging opinions and statistics. As Mom's retention of details slipped, Rick still maintained their routine as a constant in their relationship. When Mom forgot details about the game, Rick would tease her when she would say, "I'm not remembering very well anymore," or "I just can't remember like I used to."

His reply was, "Well, It's OK, Mom, because you meet new people every day and you never hear the same joke twice!" She would chuckle and smile.

The mind is really a puzzle. Mom would call periodically needing to discuss whatever was on her mind, fact or fiction. She always called my work cell phone. Busy at work, I answered whenever I could. My co-workers got a kick out of the random calls, and all I had to say was "Mom" as part of the conversation and that clarified it. I recall one time when I hung up and someone said, "It's amazing that she still remembers your phone number." Actually, that was true, of all the things that she forgot, somehow she always remembered that cell phone number. Strange. When I left that employer, I wondered who might continue to get those random phone calls, and mentioned to my manager that they may want to suggest turning it off at night.

A time came when she was anxious because she would feel like she didn't know where she was. She would call me in a panic because she "woke up somewhere else." She was very convincing during these episodes, and she would tell me she went to the store and when she came back, they had moved her. She had her own furniture at the assisted living Home, so I finally began to ask her to describe the room to me. She would still focus on the confusion and say that she had not seen any of that stuff before. They weren't her clothes in the closet; they belonged to someone else. In my emotional mind, I was still listening to my Mom having a meltdown, and she was so convincing, I half-believed her.

One of her favorite pieces of furniture from her house was a turquoise leather sectional sofa. We managed to bring one section of this sofa to the Home. If she was insistent upon the fact that she was lost or didn't know where she was, I was at an advantage here because caller ID told me where she was calling from. I would ask her if she could see her turquoise couch. When she would say, "Yes, I can," I would tell her that it meant she was in her own room. Then I would change the subject to dinner, or the weather, or something that was normal. If she cycled back to her confusion, I used the couch as the consistent reminder.

Bit by bit, pieces of the puzzle went missing forever, lost in her newfound reality void of truth and sustainable content. Keeping ahead of her was a new game as she slowly retreated from reality and me.

As Mom's illness progressed, and she was confused about the time of day, we decided to remove the phone from her apartment. She called in the middle of the night, angry because she missed lunch. "Nobody came and got me for lunch and I am hungry."

"Well, that's because it is 2 a.m., not 2 p.m., Mom." She would argue with me and I would have to say, "Mom, can you see out your window? Is it still dark outside?" "Do you have your pajamas on?"

"Well, then why am I hungry?"

In the morning, I confirmed that she had also called Rick and Dennis as if expecting a different answer.

This went on for months and we agreed that stocking the cupboards with snacks and removing the phone was the next step. If she wanted to call us, she could use the phone at the nurses' station. If it was an odd hour or a question they could help her with, they could intercept her need to make a phone call. So, as you can imagine, having the front desk as a filter for her random phone calls allowed us all to have more restful nights of sleep.

Choices have consequences, and it changed our ability to easily check in on her by calling and disconnected the pattern that she and Rick had come to rely on while watching sports. He tried to call the nurses' station and ask them to have her come to the phone, but that was often impractical since she could be roaming around just about anywhere in the facility.

Mom exhibited a lot of anger when she first moved, and at times she would refuse to eat their cooking. 'They just don't know how to cook." Mom was a fine cook and therefore had a very critical palate. Although the Home's meals were well made and a wide variety was served, the food was bland, typical of the environment and its clientele. She lost weight, and it was hard to witness the change in her eating habits, but there were only a few things I could do to influence her. Mom always liked to have a couple of cookies with some tea or her favorite international instant coffee before bed, as part of her nighttime routine. I kept a stash of her coffee choices in the small kitchenette cupboard in her room. She also loved ice cream, and although it didn't add valuable nutrition, it added a few calories. We had to cross each bridge as we came to it, and every day was a new day.

A Long, Long Time Ago

After a short time, she forgot that her mother wasn't alive any longer, as well as her siblings who had passed before her, and she would ask about them. We had several conversations when she asked us to "Go pick up Grandma in West Seattle; she's in that brick apartment on California Avenue." While listening to her description, I would try to figure out how many years back she was remembering because that was not the last apartment Grandma had lived in before she moved in with Mom and Dad. She was definitely living at least 30 years in the past.

Then came the difficult conversations of explaining to her that Grandma had died in 1988, at age 102. It was difficult because her emotional response was as if it had just happened, each time. She would say, "Grandma died?" — "How? — When?" and she would start to cry and either my brothers or I would explain it. It was sad to witness her relive the shock of the news each time it came up. Then we talked and compared our individual conversations and decided there was no point in continuing to try to explain the realities of the present as it was only upsetting her. So we decided to just change the subject or play along with the charade. We each had our own difficulties with this game as it held this underlying feeling that you were lying to your mother. It sounds strange, but I guess some aspects of ourselves and our relationships with our mother or father makes it difficult to realize that we now have become the adult in this situation and need to choose what is best for Mom. It is a shift, both mentally and emotionally.

As mentioned earlier, we siblings each had our own way of dealing with Mom's illness. Our interactions paralleled our relationship and individual bond with Mom. For instance, she and I used to go shopping together often over the years. That was our mother / daughter thing. Out to lunch and shopping; it must have started at a very early age because I cannot recall a first time for this ritual. Our favorites were Northgate Mall in Seattle, and the Grand Bazaar Kapalı Çarşı in Istanbul. Northgate, the first mall in Seattle, with its signature totem pole, eagle's wings spread wide, was only partially enclosed with covered walkways between the stores. Kapali Carsi, Turkish for Covered Bazaar, was a multitude of small shops with street-like pathways enclosed within two ancient bedestens, domes with beautifully tiled high arched ceilings. Mom and I also shared the love of animals. So if I wanted to change the focus of a conversation, (or lack of focus,) I would mention shopping, or the dog or my horses. Then we could start an entirely different conversation. This shifted the topic while it also allowed her a graceful way to escape her state of confusion.

She often became frustrated. Sometimes she would express her frustration, and sometimes it just showed on her face. It is difficult to chat with a person in an altered state of mind, and it made it hard to go visit sometimes if the previous time had been uncomfortable in any way. If she became sad and upset when I left her, I carried that experience with me and I remembered it, even though I was sure she forgot about it two minutes after I was gone. However, what I learned was that each time could be entirely different with a new challenge or experience, so on each occasion I had to arrive with an open mind and heart.

When Mom greeted me with a smile on her face and a song in her heart, the experience left me feeling that our time together had value. If the visit was a conflict of emotions, it left me feeling sad.

One day, it was as if Mom became aware that I was taking care of her like she took care of her mother. She asked for my help buttoning her blouse and as I unbuttoned it to adjust the misaligned buttoning she had attempted to do herself, she put her hand on mine and held it against her chest and looked me straight in the eye. "Thank you, Honey, I guess I can't dress myself anymore." She continued, "My arthritis hurts in my hands and now my shoulder hurts, too."

"I'm glad to help you, Mom; you know that, don't you?"

She replied with a slight smile, "Yes, Honey, and I love you for it!"

This touched my heart. I finished buttoning her blouse and distracted myself by saying, "Want to go see if they are still serving ice cream sundaes in the lunchroom?" as I helped her up and slid her walker in front of her.

Dennis' and Mom's connection was all about music. Dennis was a drummer in many bands over the years and Mom enjoyed watching him perform. She sewed the band's fancy satin dress shirts and offered her living room for combo practice one or two nights a week. I remember being sent to bed early in hopes that I would be asleep before they started playing. Considering that my bedroom was next to the living room, it was inevitable that I would be awakened and get into trouble for dancing on my bed.

Dennis and Mom liked the same styles of music and he would bring her CD's to share. When he took Mom to her doctor appointments, they would ride in the car together listening to blues or anything with a good rhythm. She would sing along while Dennis played the drums on the steering wheel and dash board.

Rick was the athletic one in the family and his connection with Mom was anything sports! They watched games together, tracked draft picks and even watched from different locations while badgering referees and cheering through a telephone.

As the illness progressed, she retreated further back in time in her memories. She worked for the telephone company as an operator for "Ma Bell"

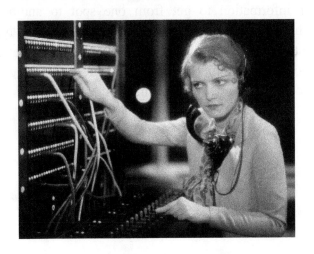

long before I was born. She was one of those old-time operators who connected each call manually, while wearing a headset with a group of wires plugged into a switchboard. A real switchboard. Mom answered the phone, "Operator, may I help you?" Then she would plug in a wire to complete the circuit and say, "You are connected."

I always have wondered if they really did listen in on those calls, or if they had a choice. During one of our conversations, she said she was "late for work" and "my boss is going to be upset, because the board isn't covered." It took me a while to connect those dots, or wires. That thought created an image for me. It helped me to visualize what was going on inside that brain of hers. If the brain is a series of connections, then there is a wire, similar to the old switchboard, for information to get from one spot to another. When it was unplugged, it was just unplugged. No matter what you said or did, you would not get a good connection. But once the wire was plugged back in, there you were again: "You are connected."

Visiting Dementia Land

My brothers and I had our own routines, but each of us would go see Mom at different times to maintain a semi-reliable frequency. We rarely were there at the same time unless invited by the Home to a group meal, patient conference or event. We realized that we needed to keep each other appraised of the status of our independent visits and started sending out group emails to one another, with updates.

As far as the transition to her new home and her memory issues went, she fit nicely in and made new friends. The staff tried to impose an informal, safe yet accessible environment as much as possible and the residents had some freedom to roam the facility on the lower two floors. The third floor was secured and a code was necessary to get onto or off the elevator on that floor. Mom kept trying to leave the building because she thought she needed to go to work or to the grocery store. She broke out a few too many times, and as her condition worsened it was recommended that, for her own safety, she reside on the secured floor. This occurred during the second year in the progression of her dementia.

Emotions are something we all try to control as any illness progresses, but I had a really hard time with the lockdown transition. It felt like we were putting our mother in jail, since I needed a security code to get off the elevator. I found it more and more difficult to go to see her.

When Mom lived on the second floor, I established a pattern of going on weekends. After lock up, I noticed that I felt anxious for days prior to visiting and it became stressful for me. I found it was easier to either take someone with me, or go after work during dinnertime. Bringing my dinner with me and sitting together with Mom's group of friends in the dining room helped. I guess it also had something to do with the fact that group conversation was generic and became a distraction for me from my newfound reality. It took me a while to get over my own fears and force myself into a new routine. Once I did, it was easier.

I traveled with my job over these two years, so when I was away I would send postcards from the various cities I was in. This also helped the staff to remind her that her daughter was in Nashville, Las Vegas or wherever the card was from. When I returned, we would look at the postcards and talk about my trips.

One night when I arrived, Mom was right there staring at the door as its latch clicked open when I entered the four digit code. She looked and sounded angry. "Thank God you're here to take me home," she exclaimed. "For crying-out-loud, they won't tell me how to get this damn door open!"

I smiled a forced smile, and said "Hi, Mom. How are you?"

"Mad!" I thought she was mad at me and, combined with my guilt and anxiety, I was uneasy and near tears. The voice of reason inside me said, "Crying isn't going to help here, so put on your big girl pants and deal with it!" Sometimes I hate my voice of reason.

Conversations with the demented mind are a challenge. There were times, when she didn't know what time of day it was, or if I had just arrived or had just left and come back. Sometimes I would arrive, we would say our greetings, talk a bit and then she would need to use the restroom. When finished, she would come out and say, "Well look who the cat dragged in. When did you get here?" Mom had always been sarcastic and dealt with life using a graceful, humorous glamour. It was comforting that the dementia never seemed to affect that portion of her brain. We would visit, and she would always ask me how work was; that became a new pattern that seemed to work well for us. Mom worked until she was in her 80's and therefore she always honored work commitments.

Because she loved animals and had various pets over the years, she was true to those commitments, too. Somehow, some way, even if she didn't remember where I worked or where I lived, it was easy to talk about work, or the horses or the dog, because the topic was familiar.

Mom was a big flirt and could easily strike up a conversation with anyone, so I had teased her about going out man shopping with me as she would make a great wing man. She laughed and reminded me that she was a widow now and she needed a man, too! We agreed she could pick a cute guy and we would team up on him and maybe we both could get lucky! Greeting Mom was always easy for that very reason, but on this day she was not responsive. She was sitting in the dining hall and appeared deep in thought; as I greeted her she barely looked up at me. So, I asked if she wanted some tea and she just nodded yes. I went to the counter and made two cups of tea, grabbed two sugars for hers and came back to the table. *Maybe she'll forget I was here and I can try this again*, I thought. "Hi, Mom. Would you like some tea?"

"Yes." No other acknowledgement or response, just yes.

Knowing that her arthritis was progressively

causing more pain, I opened her sugar and handed them to her. "How was your morning?"

"Boring."

Well Ok then, I thought, *we're in a bit of a mood today.* "What did you have for breakfast?"

Squinting as if thinking was difficult today, "I don't remember."

I could continue to probe answers out of her, or just ignore her mood and tell her about my normal day, so I did. I complained about the traffic, talked about the weather, told her I painted the house, her house, thinking maybe that would spark some sort of interest.

Nothing, absolutely nothing familiar about this. *Where did she go when she disappeared in that mind of hers? Who is this moody sulking person across the table from me?*

I went back to the kitchen counter to ask the staff if they had noticed anything wrong. They explained that on occasion, Mom just got quiet and then either a little later on or the next day she would be herself again. *I certainly hope so* I thought, *this could get old really fast! I know I don't have the patience for this.*

We made it through another cup of tea and I hugged her, gave her a peck on the cheek and excused myself, telling her I needed to pick up dog food and I would be back soon.

I tried to understand her mood and while considering her adventurous spirit, being there in that place would be a very boring existence for anyone, particularly Mom.

As conversations gradually became more and more of a challenge, I would turn on the TV and we could talk about the present. She maintained a quick wit about the present. She would speak excitedly about something, yet using words that did not belong together in a sentence. Response was nearly impossible. BJ's experience with Mary Jean came in handy and she compared these experiences with a young child that you cannot understand, when just acknowledging with a nod and a smile was enough. The mind is truly a puzzle, and I came to the conclusion that it didn't need to make sense to me, as long as being there made her happy. It's Dementia Land, after all and I encourage you to try your damndest to become the adult, however difficult it is, and just go with the flow.

Departures became more difficult. She would beg me not to leave. She threw a crying, sobbing tantrum with Rick once, and it was really hard for him. It caused a natural apprehension for him to return. However, one thing became apparent; each visit was unique, as she was always in a different place and time. Therefore, departure was an ever-changing experience. With experimentation in various exit strategies, I came up with some solutions that worked for me. In order to make the 'routine' of my departure easier for both of us, I learned that if I took her to the kitchen area and asked them to make her a hot chocolate, then she would be with others, rather than alone in her room, when I left her. Since she didn't understand that I wasn't coming back, I could tell her I needed to go to work, or go feed the dog, or go to the grocery store. Those were all things that she could relate to, and they helped.

When she asked if she could come with me, I had to think on my feet and come up with a believable reason why she couldn't. She would miss her favorite TV show, her exercise class or the ice cream social. I had to learn how to fib to my mother. It was unbelievably hard to do, but in this case it felt like it was the right thing given the circumstances. Still, the underlying rule about 'Don't ever lie to your mother', haunted my subconscious every time I told her I would be right back, or any other stretching of the truth.

The lesson I learned here was about being okay with

what had to be done and not send myself on a guilt trip. It is a tough place to be in life and my heart goes out to you if you are heading down this path. Please know that most have survived the emotion, the struggles and feel better for participating in the journey.

Most people are glad they did not hide from it. It would have been easy to be too busy, too tired, or any number of excuses, but I had to stop and think that Mom was always there for me under all those same conditions. After all, it is a true test of unconditional love, loving someone who isn't the person you once knew and admired. They still need our love, regardless of their present state of mind.

The simple truth; there were times when I just could not make myself go. I justified it by thinking I had too much to do it all or other commitments, when it was just fear talking. If I had that little chat with myself, that she wasn't going to be here forever and could I live with myself if I chose not to go, then I booted my butt out of my little pity party. I decided that Sundays were the best day of the week for me and just did it. Sundays, still and forever, will remind me of my visits with Mom with a happy heart and no regrets.

Outings

Mom loved musicals and performing, so I took her out to a live performance when the schedule allowed. As time and her mental state progressed, it became too hard for her to leave and come back, because it just made her more confused.

She was a performer. Not only was she always the center of attention in any situation, she tap danced until she was 87. She was accustomed to being on stage and loved it. Lynne and I took her to a performance at a local theater, and when I called to purchase the tickets and arranged for wheelchair seating to simplify the experience, I mentioned her performance history to the manager. When we arrived, we were greeted and escorted to our seats by the manager. She told me that, if Mom felt like it, after the performance we could take her backstage as a special treat. Just let her know, she said, and she would meet us by the backstage entrance. I assumed that Mom would love this special attention and looked forward to the experience.

Mom enjoyed the dancing and singing, tapped her feet to the rhythm and applauded at all the appropriate times. After the show, we met the manager by the backstage door. Mom became very confused and couldn't understand why we turned left through the door labeled 'STAGE' in big bold letters, instead of exiting with all the other people. She firmly planted her feet on the floor and was trying to stop the wheelchair from moving. "Stop! This is not the right way," she yelled. She still looked frightened after I explained again that we were getting a special treat, a backstage pass. I began to wonder if this was as good an idea as we had intended it to be.

Of course! She saw only strangers in front of her; Lynne and I were both behind the wheelchair. When Lynne went ahead and walked in front of Mom and talked to her, Mom calmed down and let the chair roll freely.

The manager was gracious and patiently described in detail each area we passed – the stage, the green room, stage sets that might remind Mom of her past trouping experiences. Our efforts did not have their desired effect. She became more fearful backstage, so we thanked the manager and told Mom we would leave any time she wanted to. That calmed and soothed her, and she relaxed.

I suppose Lynne and I were hoping to bring the past back into the present for us as much as for Mom. I soon felt like I had lost another part of my mother and I would miss that unique part of our life together. I reflected back on many events we had attended together, on the fun times we had choosing what to wear, getting ready, going out to dinner and talking about the show as we drove home. Another part of our journey had become a memory that only I could hold in my heart.

Ivar's clam chowder was her favorite and there was one of the fast food style restaurants within blocks of the Home, so we would often go out for lunch. She always ordered the same senior meal. All of us took her there, so with her frequent lunch dates, the clerks got to know her and they were all welcoming and attentive. She liked the attention; that soon became part of the fun. They even knew what she ordered which was helpful when she forgot herself, but she was always happy to be served. When they delivered her Two Piece Fish and Chips with Chowder meal to the table, she would always ask with a smile: "How did you know that is my favorite?" Over time, this became routine to me, yet she seemed to enjoy each lunch as if it was a new experience.

I pondered the thought of our déjà vu experience as if we were in a continual rerun loop that might vary with only the slightest seasonal change. Yet what was a déjà vu for me was apparently a new experience for Mom.

She loved to shop, so I would take her to the store in her wheelchair and we would roam the racks of clothes, just like old times. For most of my life, Mom had worked in the world of retail. She was responsible for balancing all the tills and scheduling staff and over the years she developed many good friendships with her colleagues. The familiarity of racks of clothes seemed comforting to her. She would look at the prices and ask me, "I hope they'll still give me my discount; I don't have my badge with me." Occasionally we would find something she liked and I would have to decide if it was something she really needed or simply move on to the next department hoping she would forget about the green sweater that looked just like one she already had.

Even when I didn't take her out shopping with me, I tried to bring her some of her favorites, a new sweater or a magazine; chocolate was always a hit, and flowers were, too.

The Christmas Eve Tradition

When I purchased Mom's house, the Christmas traditions naturally fell on my shoulders. Since it was the home in which all three generations had grown up, I honored the Christmas Eve at Grandma's house tradition by hosting the family festivities.

I was nervous the first time she came as I had made several changes to her house. The first was to rip up the gold shag carpet and refinish the fir floors. I was pleased with them, and I knew that though they had lived in the house for over 60 years, she must have had bare floors at some point. I also removed the beloved floor to ceiling draperies. She liked the changes and it didn't present any new anxiety for her. She even complimented what I had done. To all intents and purposes, I believe she remembered the way it was before, even though I will never really know for sure.

Mom seemed to enjoy herself and everything went well, but she did exhibit some slight confusion. Although we tried to get her to sit and relax with family, she felt more at home in the kitchen while BJ and I were cooking. In the confines of a very small kitchen, we managed to maneuver around and get dinner on the table. When she started opening cupboards looking for her own dishes, we distracted her by giving her something to do. She had trouble navigating with her cane or walker and the bathroom was up four steps, so Dennis set up a portable potty, originally from his camper, in the den. He had set it up on some lumber to raise it to a comfortable sitting level for Mom, and it worked.

This was so typical of how we all managed our lives, as Mom would say, 'we jury rigged' this and that to make it work. Dennis showed her where it was, and she used it a couple of times with assistance. We anticipated one of her sarcastic comments about remodeling her den into a bathroom, but she was just confused enough with all the festivities that she didn't seem to care where it was.

As the evening progressed, we were attentive to her, and yet while we were dishing up the food, we didn't notice when she said she had to go to the bathroom. She decided to go up the stairs to the bathroom, entirely forgetting about the porta potty in the den. My nephew, Bear, helped her up the stairs and then she became distracted and went towards her old bedroom, now mine.

She began going through the closet, saying she was looking for something. Bear, who was accustomed to following his Grandma's wishes, found himself faced with a bit of a challenge on his hands. From downstairs, I heard all the commotion and overheard that she wanted to know what I had done with all her clothes? BJ and I raced up the stairs to find Mom standing in front of my closet with doors wide open, pulling clothes out and tossing them on my bed. Bear shrugged and said, "She won't listen to me and wants to know what you did with all her clothes!" BJ, a fourth grade teacher for 30 years, handled Mom like a peach and talked her back into using the bathroom. Mom gave me her shame-on-you look as she walked past me, escorted on BJ's arm.

It became obvious that she was sundowning as the evening progressed. Sundowner's Syndrome describes the increased confusion in dementia patients at twilight and beyond. Ask anyone who has worked in a nursing home. No matter the reason for the patients' admittance, everyone seems to become more confused around dinnertime and beyond. Any explanation I offered regarding my clothes in her closet was pointless.

As we were cleaning up the dinner dishes before opening gifts, Mom, my other nephew, Gregg, and I were all in the kitchen. Mom announced, "I have a question. I am trying to figure out how you two are related." Then she proceeded with, "Are you her brother?"

"No, because that would make you my mother," Gregg joked.

Mom had a very puzzled look on her face and said, "Well that can't be, because I am your Grandma." We tried to explain that I was his aunt and he was my brother Dennis' son, along with who was related to whom and spelled out the family tree as best we could. She still appeared confused and eventually changed the subject by saying "Well, that's enough about that!" Avoidance became a skilled behavior when she realized she was confused to the point that she couldn't find her way out. She could have a conversation about the present moment with wit and ease, but at times, reflection on the past presented a struggle for her.

The next Christmas, she was in a wheelchair and it was easier to keep her on the main floor. It had snowed on this Christmas Eve, uncommon for Western Washington, and it presented travel challenges. Driving was treacherous, let alone maneuvering a wheel chair in the snow, but it was fun for all of us to be together. A high point occurred at the end of the evening, when Dennis had to stop down the road and put chains on his truck to get up the hill. Mom was so cute, sitting in the back seat of his big Ford 350

Quadcab, just patiently waiting. Sam and I went to help and when I opened the door to check on her and explain what we were doing, she asked, "Do I need to get out and push?" A happy memory.

The Neighborhood Brunch

It was summer, and her friends that we had met at the restaurant after church, invited us for Sunday brunch at their house. I thought it would be nice for Mom to revisit the neighborhood again in the summertime. When I arrived at the Home, she was in her room all dressed with a variety of bright colors and she had something in her hair. One of the staff came in just as I asked, "Mom, what did you put in your hair?"

"Nothing," she answered.

"Mom, you have something pink in your hair; what is it?" I told her, "You look like a punk rocker." I searched her dresser for whatever was pink, as she looked in her small handheld mirror. She couldn't see much with the shades drawn.

She insisted "I don't see anything; there is nothing in my hair!" and she added, "And we better get going or we'll be late." I coaxed her to walk with her cane toward the bathroom with a big brightly lit mirror, which took a little while as age was one step ahead of her dance shoes these days. "What is all that pink stuff in my hair," she wailed.

The aide tried hard not to laugh out loud. I said, "Mom, it looks like lipstick; why did you put pink lipstick in your hair?" She insisted she didn't; it was hair gel to make her curl stay put. The aide apologized and said she had just given Mom a shower and got her dressed, but left her alone to put on her makeup. It certainly wasn't the aide's fault, but there just wasn't enough time to wash Mom's hair. We either had to cancel, or go as is. We tried to comb it out, but it just wasn't going to come out without a good thorough washing.

In her defense, the lighting in her mini apartment wasn't that great when the sun wasn't shining through the windows. Many times, she would close the drapes for privacy. I never understood that change, because she was always one to enjoy any view through a window with lots of daylight. I thought she had chosen this room for its nice view of a greenbelt and no adjacent buildings, but apparently that changed, too.

I opted to go, since they were very good friends and would understand. So I called ahead and warned them. "You will understand this better when we get there, but please don't mention anything about her hair." Cory said he would let everyone know.

When we arrived, they were all smiles and greeted her affectionately, "Oh it is so good to see you Corrine!" We kept her away from the bathroom mirror and she had a wonderful time with her friends. It was just one of those times when it was best to hide from the truth.

On another occasion, I arrived and she had green eyebrows. I asked her where her makeup was and she pointed to the dresser. I asked if I could help her with her makeup and cleaned the green eyeliner off and put brown eyebrows on. She never left the house without her 'face on,' as she put it. A beautiful woman, she always looked her best. This struck my heart like a bolt of lightning, but I felt I needed to leave her with a limited supply of makeup so that she could look presentable no matter what. I left mascara, brown eyebrow pencil, blush and lipstick in hopes that they would wind up in the right place on her face. No more eye shadows that could be put on her cheekbones or colored eyeliner that could be put on her brows. I was saddened to realize that she had arrived in this place in her life.

This Home specialized in Memory Care. They had decorated the facility quite nicely with furniture, paintings of the time period for the ages of the clientele. One hallway had photos of actors famous from their generation. Clark Gable, Gregory Peck, Marilyn Monroe, and Elvis Presley, Mom's favorite. Whenever we walked past the Elvis Presley photo, she would tell her story about Elvis Presley at the

World's Fair. In 1962 when Seattle held the world's fair, Elvis Presley made a movie and Mom and a couple of her friends had signed up to be extras in the movie. As Mom would tell it, she and Elvis hit it off and had lunch together one day. Those were fond memories for her that she never forgot, and they always brought a smile to her face. She also complained that in the movie, as she was pitching pennies into a fountain standing behind Elvis, her slip was showing from under her skirt. I always reassured her, that I'm sure no one else noticed her slip as they were busy watching Elvis.

One quaint little sitting room near the elevator was made up like a little wedding chapel with an old wedding dress hanging on a hook. The main dining room set the tables with white linen tablecloths and nice table settings like a semi-formal restaurant. The Home served coffee in a cup and saucer instead of a mug. They made every effort to create a familiar environment for their residents.

Religion

A small chapel at the Home invited the residents to go and sit, pray or just listen to the soft gospel music. Some of them would say grace at their group tables in the dining hall and each person's religious individuality was respected. At some point, while eating lunch, there was a discussion amongst a few about their beliefs and where they attended church in the past. In general, the topic did not usually generate any disputes, however one particular day it did.

Mom was very proud of her fifty years with her Presbyterian Church and apparently mentioned her preferred denomination to the group. Another woman had very strong feelings about the Presbyterian religion and voiced her concerns directed at Mom, who took it personally. They argued. The staff tried to calm the situation and made certain their lunch schedules did not place them together at the same table. Mom recited the conflict repeatedly when we spoke on the phone and openly expressed her frustration with it and referred to her religious opponent as 'That Woman.'

One day I arrived in time to join her for lunch in the dining room. We sat and caught up while enjoying lunch together. The table settings were elegant with linens, china and flowers and it really did feel like we were dining out at a restaurant. After lunch, we left the dining room and headed back towards her private room. While we were waiting for the elevator and chatting, the elevator door opened and I entered. As I held the door with one hand and reached out to help Mom with the other, her face was stern, devoid of her usual smile. She waved her cane firmly and with purpose. *Now what,* I thought. *Is she afraid of the elevator again,* and I said aloud, "Come on, Mom, we're going up to your room, remember?"

She said, "No, I am not going!" I was getting used to her patterns of confusion, but tried again, telling her I'd help her into the elevator car. She spoke very deliberately and said, "I am NOT getting in that elevator with HER," raising her cane in the air again. There were two people in the elevator and, I was embarrassed with her behavior and attitude. I backed out, saying "Sorry, I guess we'll catch the next one." The other woman stood firm with her hands on her hips and a smug look in her eye, watching the elevator door close.

I looked at Mom with that shame-on-you look that she often threw my way and before I could say anything, she said, "I don't like her." I told her she wasn't acting like herself at all, thinking, *Children, these two gray haired women are behaving just like children!*

Mom began to describe, word for word, every detail from their point of conflict, how she always has to look out for her in the hallways and how mean she has been to her. I realized this was 'That Woman' and as I listened, as usual I had my own puzzling thoughts running through my head. *How is it that she wouldn't remember if we were coming from the dining room, or on our way to eat, but she can replay this moment from over a month ago, word for word and filled with all the emotions as if it had just happened?*

She simply had locked in her anger and stored it in a location in her brain that allowed instant and total recall. As I understand it, when we experience something of significant emotional impact, the brain has the ability to recall more details after the fact than a normal day to day event. It makes sense, and her recall of this hurtful experience was proof enough for me.

It was also one of those situations where I instantly knew that I was the parent and she was the child. That feeling is incredibly hard to get used to.

Teeth

The next heartache was her teeth. She had several bridges and false upper teeth and very few of her own teeth remained at this time of her life. She complained that her teeth sometimes bothered her. Dennis often took her to the dentist, who said the real problem was due to her inconsistently wearing them. When they rubbed and felt uncomfortable, she would take them out as soon as she finished her meal because they hurt. As I understand it now, you need to build up calluses on your gums and she had removed them so often, the calluses were gone and the teeth were uncomfortable.

So, she repeatedly lost and found her teeth, how many times no one knows, but in the end she wrapped them in a napkin and laid them on her dining tray and they were lost for good. I had watched her wrap them as she was tidying up her meal tray and although I tried reminding her many times, it went in one ear and out the other. We replaced them once, to the tune of nearly $3000, but again they were lost. It became apparent that the simplest solution was pureeing her food for her. This had its own issues, but my challenge was getting used to seeing Mom without her teeth. The woman that would never leave the house without her makeup, perfectly coifed hair and beautiful smile, was now without her teeth. It broke my heart. *This will haunt me 'til the day I die,* I thought. And it does.

Unbeknownst to us, at the time that we were solving one problem with the teeth, we created another. Mom was a great cook and as a result, very cuisine oriented. I had several meals at the Home, and their chefs should be complimented for their selection and seasoning. Earlier you said the food was very bland. Which is it: seasoned high end food or bland cafeteria food? It was just like eating in a high end restaurant. Mom no longer liked the food, because it was pureed. She would taste what was offered to her, but politely say, "No thank you," constantly leaving her plate without eating enough. I don't know if I could bring myself to eat spaghetti and meatballs if they were a soup, either. You would think they would taste the same but texture and independent flavors do have something to do with our appreciation for the food we eat. If we fed her, she eventually accepted small bites. Although she was certainly capable of feeding herself, she just wouldn't. The staff was wonderful and tried to get her to eat more pureed solid foods, but we resorted to liquid nutritional meal replacements to sustain her. She lived on Ensure for two years. We all continued to attempt to get her to eat the pureed foods and she would eat ice cream, puddings and such, but not consistently from the more nutritious selections.

Doctor Appointments and Illnesses

Dennis managed Mom's medications and most of her doctors' appointments; as Mom said, they "would make a day of it." She had a good relationship with her physician and he was very cognizant of her need for attention. He enjoyed her humor and wit, and was just as witty with his comments to her; it was always a positive experience. As her illness progressed, even though she was obviously confused, the privacy issues that medical practices have to respect resulted in the need for documentation to allow family to participate. When I took her, she had to sign a form stating that they could release information to me. With all the HIPAA (Health Insurance Portability and Accountability Act) laws in place, eventually Dennis had to use the power of attorney rights and could sit in during the exam and ask the questions. She obviously wasn't going to remember what the doctor told her, so this was a critical part of her ongoing care. Then, because she would forget what the doctor said, when we had to remind her, family became the messenger, usually of something she did not want to do.

One of the times when Mom needed to have some medical tests, she had become anxious and confused upon leaving the Home and not knowing where we were going. So, because this appointment was involving some tests that might be uncomfortable for her, the doctor prescribed a mild sedative. I picked her up, put the wheelchair in the back of a car and we ventured downtown to Virginia Mason Hospital. I gave her one of her prescribed pills twenty minutes before the appointment as directed.

Her appointment was in the radiology department where there was a very large waiting room with a fish tank. We arrived early, checked in at the desk and then seated ourselves along the wall so we could watch the fish. Mom was always one to strike up conversations with strangers, so it didn't surprise me when she started talking to the elderly gentleman sitting next to her. They quickly learned that they both attended the same high school, West Seattle High. Mom's mild sedative seemed to have kicked in and she was getting a little giddy. The waiting room, filled with 15 to 20 people, was in for a treat. Mom and her new friend were both joyfully singing their high school song. The entire waiting room listened and laughed with them as they reminisced about their high school days. I couldn't help myself and I asked Mom what kind of pills the doctor gave her, because I'd like one, too. We all joined in laughter and I believe it broke the ice for many people awaiting their own radiology appointments.

When they called her name, Mom announced to the

whole group, "It's my turn," slowly squaring herself into her wheelchair, "y'all will just have to wait for the next show!" Her social skills and humor seemed to survive even her most difficult days with dementia. And unbeknownst to her, she helped us all get through this and many other difficult times. As I sat alone and waited for her procedure to finish I thought, *how can she remember her high school song like it was yesterday when I can't even remember mine?*

The very independent nature of my mother caused its own problems. She would forget she was supposed to use her walker, or cane, leaving it behind in the cafeteria or restroom. She eventually fell and broke her hip while in the assisted living facility and needed reconstructive hip surgery. Following her hip surgery, she went to rehabilitation. Again, following directions, reminding her of her care needs became even more complicated in Dementia Land.

How Mom broke her hip became more confusing every time she told me the story. It has never been clear in my mind what actually happened that day. She told me a story about mopping the floor and while she was mopping the floor, she dumped the bucket over and then slipped, landing on her left side by the door. The only part of that that seemed true was that she remembered landing on her left side by the door, which is where the aides found her when they heard her cry for help. It has never made sense to me how she could come up with the whole story about mopping the floor, other than she didn't really know how she fell so she just made it up. Of course, when she started telling the doctors this story there was some initial concern about safety in the Home, but it soon became apparent that she was in a constant state of confusion. The reports from the Home were well documented and neither Dennis nor Rick were concerned that there was any reason to doubt them. I was out of town at the time when Dennis called, and I contemplated returning home, torn between Mom and the training that I had waited for quite some time to attend. Dennis and Rick reassured me that they could handle it, and they did. They decided that the Home was okay, but Mom was not.

I called the hospital to talk to Mom and see how she was feeling. Rick answered the phone by her bed. "Hello, Corrine's not talking today, this is Rick, what can I do you for?"

"Hi, it's me, how's Mom?"

He snorted, "I don't know because she isn't talking today."

"What do you mean she isn't talking; what's wrong?" I asked.

"She wouldn't talk to Dennis, so he and Donna left to go get lunch. We thought maybe if I just stayed here with her, she might cooperate a little more." He continued. "Which isn't the case. Her lips are clinched together like she is mad and she barely talks to the nurses, only answered their questions after we told her that she had to cooperate."

I thought maybe the phone could fake her out of it. "Well, hand her the phone and see if she'll talk to me." She didn't say anything and I could barely hear her breathing. "Mom, it's Faith, are you okay?"

Softly she said, "No, where are you?" Her voice was raspy.

"I am still in Nashville for training. How are you feeling? Is your throat sore from the surgery?"

"Yes," she whispered.

"Well, I won't make you talk, then. I will be home on Friday and see you then. I love you and I miss you, Mom."

I couldn't understand what she said, but she handed

the phone back to Rick who said, "I've been sitting here all day trying to get her to talk and you're the one who's not here and she's mad at me!"

"Well, you know how stubborn she can be, but she didn't really have a choice with a phone now, did she? I think she has a sore throat; better ask the nurse for a lozenge. I need to get back into class, break is over. Call me if anything changes, I love you."

As we hung up, I heard him saying to Mom, "I thought I was your favorite."

I returned Friday as promised and she had been discharged from the hospital and moved to a rehabilitation facility. The layout of the facility was like a traditional nursing home, with a nurse's station across the hall. Mom was all settled in a room with a roommate and seemed pleased to see me. She, however said, "Good you can take me home, I don't know where I am or why I woke up here."

While in rehab, Mom was to do daily exercises under the guidance of the staff physical therapist. They had posted the same note in several places in Mom's room to remind her. The signs read, "Do not cross your legs," which Mom had done ever since I can remember. When Mom read the sign out loud to me and asked, "Why can't I cross my legs?" I explained that she had hip replacement surgery and that was why she had to do the exercises. She looked puzzled and said, "I had hip surgery? Why?" I don't know why this surprised me, but each time I explained, each time she forgot, so this time I reached over and pulled the top of her pants down just enough to uncover the scar along her left hip. As she started to object grabbing hold of her pants and asking, "What are you…," interrupting herself, "Where did that come from?" as she looked more closely at her leg. Somehow, this time it stuck because she had a visual reference to add to the memory. The next thing I knew, she was telling people she had a new hip and maybe she could dance again.

When she changed residences, the new staff was unfamiliar with her demented condition. Because she often appeared quite lucid, they assumed she could make her own decisions. We had to seek documentation from her doctors to be sure we could help making decisions regarding her care protocol. I would highly recommend anyone in this predicament to get a thorough physical and mental exam for your loved one so you have documentation proving competence or incompetence for the safety and security of yourselves and your loved one.

NeuroPsychiatric Evaluation

As part of Mom's care plan, it was decided to have a neuropsychiatric evaluation. Mom had the personality and grace to charm her way through the exam but since it was so thorough, she could not hide even the slightest evidence of memory loss. The evaluation was an interesting process and done so well that Mom just felt like she was being interviewed. Over the course of these six years she had two cognitive neuro-psych evaluations. The first one, prior to Dad's passing, was used as a baseline; the second test showed the advanced progression of her illness. The evaluation consisted of a series of questions that were presented in a conversational style interview. It was a comfortable way for her to discuss her life's memories and the questions were very effective in comparing past and present. Mom loved to talk and it was like show and tell and story time for her, so in her case this was easy. She attempted to dance her way through the session with humor when she was unable to answer. When asked who the current president of the United States was, she paused and enthusiastically responded, "Me!" The results were a diagnosis that helped us to face the reality of the situation.

As Mom's six weeks of rehab progressed, she

gradually became more cooperative and fond of her new surroundings. We met with Mom's social worker, physical therapist and doctor to discuss the next phase of care. It was determined that she really needed 24 hour supervision and the previous assisted living environment was not going to be enough care for her any longer. We arranged for a tour of the onsite, 24 hour, full care resident's wing within the same building. The full time resident's wing was under the same management and staff now familiar to all of us. Since we were all pleased with the care Mom had received while at the rehab facility, we decided to put her name on the waiting list. A room just around the corner soon became available and she transitioned nicely into that new permanent living situation. Her roommate, Helga, a sweet retired hairdresser with a Norse accent made the same transition and they were roommates for the duration of her care.

The rooms were set up as a traditional nursing home, with two resident beds per room. This room, painted soft yellow with a colorful floral patterned wallpaper border, had a bay window view of the garden court. Helga chose the side of the room with the bay window, and Mom chose the bed closest to the door. Each bed faced its own closet vanity with a mirror and a spot for a TV. A floral print curtain could be pulled for privacy between beds as needed. In the corner by the door, there was a private bathroom with an accessible shower down the hall.

Now we had to move her personal furniture and belongings from the mini apartment at the assisted living Home, because all she needed here were her clothes, a few personal items and TV. There went the assistance of the familiar turquoise couch I had used as a reference point on so many occasions.

We packed up the apartment and Dennis and Rick moved everything to Mom's storage unit near Dennis' house. When she asked for the occasional clothing item or book, Dennis retrieved them for her. Although we realized now that she resided in a traditional nursing home, and would not need her furniture any longer, we didn't feel that we could just toss out her life's belongings while she still lived.

Confusion For Both Of Us

I used to just bring Mom over to my house so we could spend time together. I would do a day of laundry and cleaning while she kept me company. She watched her shows and I found it was easier for both of us when the environment resembled a familiar lifestyle and routines. Easier for me because not only could I stay busy, but my chores were distractions from the conversations that confused me. Yes, in her demented state, she confused me. I found it hard to follow her train of thought. I'm not sure I ever got over that while in the midst of it.

I still hoped that Mom could be fixed. I believe that we all tend to maintain a sense of hope throughout each situation life presents. So, when there isn't a solution, learning to cope can be one of the most difficult challenges we have to face as the realities of day-to-day life unfolds.

On one day, I made one of her favorites, homemade split pea soup. We sat down at the table together and ate our soup and crackers. She always put butter on her saltine crackers and ate several this time. I finished my soup first and asked if she wanted seconds. She said, "Not now thank you, I'm full." She gave me 'that look' when I returned with my second bowl and announced, "That is rude, young lady!"

I said, "What is, Mom?" She informed me that I had not given her anything to eat and here I was eating in front of her without offering her any soup. I tried to convince her that she refused seconds and that is why she wasn't eating anything.

"I have not had anything to eat," she insisted.

I looked at her empty bowl and asked, "Well then, who ate all that?"

She continued to insist that she had not eaten it. I wondered: *after a bowl of soup and all those crackers, you don't even feel slightly full? How can I argue with this?* She was so insistent and getting angry, so all I could do was apologize and get her some more soup. These situations were frustrating for me. I was looking for logic in the illogical world of dementia. It was hard to not express my frustration and it was also hard to accept the inevitable changes as they presented themselves, one by one.

This situation reminded me of one of the early signs back when she still lived at home, when she called me, sniffling and crying. I was concerned and asked what had upset her. She said that she had just watched the final episode of MASH, and was sad because it was one of her favorite shows and she wouldn't be able to see it anymore. "Don't worry about it, Mom," I said. "I'll get you the season recording and you can watch it as much as you want." MASH had already been in reruns for two decades.

TV, in general, had the effect of rebooting Mom's memory and I used it to do just that. There were TV shows that were her favorites, and I recorded them so that when she came over I could start one and use it to orient her back to normal. Or so I thought. She loved Matlock and MASH. If she was in front of a TV and watching something familiar she became more comfortable, and the familiarity seemed to calm her. When she was calm, I was calm.

When she was comfortable, she also became less likely to demand that she wanted to go back home. When she said "I want to go home," she was thinking of the house where she lived for over 60 years, and not the Home she had recently become accustomed to, the one she often insisted her children had stuck her in. Thus, taking her back to her various residences was a problem. She would get upset when I returned her to the 'wrong house!' Especially if it was the end of the day, when she was sundowning. As time went on, time away from

'The Home' became more challenging and turned into holiday excursions only.

I was feeling more confused by her confusion. *When she was at the nursing home, she asked to "go home," and meant her old house. Yet while we were at her old house, sitting at her beloved claw foot antique oak dining table eating our soup, she asked to "go home." Wasn't she already there?* I concluded that it was the best way for her to say, "I am tired and I want to leave."

What Did She Just Say?

My Mom was half German and although my Grandma didn't speak German often, she must have done so when Mom was younger. I don't ever recall hearing my Mom speak more than just a few words in German or the lyrics of a song she sang to us as children. As her dementia progressed, and her short term memory was a distant thought, she began to bring up things further and further in her past. Early on in the rehab phase following her hip surgery, I went to see her and found her out in the hall with her new friend, Helga. As I walked down the hall, I was so happy to see them talking and laughing, and they really seemed to be having fun. As I got close enough to hear, I realized that they were not speaking English at all, and having a grand old time. Mom would say something, Helga would respond and then they both laughed. The amused nurse told me they had been carrying on like this for quite a while, but she couldn't understand a word they said.

Shortly after, Helga's daughter came to visit, and I told her all about our mothers' lengthy conversation in German. "Mom doesn't speak German, but she speaks Norwegian," the daughter told me. We had a laugh when we realized that although they were having a fabulous conversation, neither one must have understood what the other was saying! *I replayed this incident so many times in my head, again trying to analyze the demented mind, and the only thing that made sense to me was that they were like children playing in a world of make-believe that we really didn't need to understand.*

As time went on, one of the aides would speak to Mom in German and they would have their own little sing-along of songs that I had no idea Mom even knew. She was so far back in time, it was before I was even born! *How was that possible, given all the years in between? It seemed the demented mind could remember what the normal mind could not.*

"Hi, Mom, how was your day?" I asked as I pulled a chair up close to her. Her chair was turned facing the window, her elbows on the windowsill as she stared down across the trees in the alley below. As I sat down next to her, she looked up at me without expression and then back at the view without acknowledgment that I was anyone other than one of the staff. I waited in wonder; had she already arrived at that point in the journey when she didn't know me? I too, disappeared as I stared out the window thinking deep thoughts when Holly, one of the staff, greeted me and asked if we would like some tea.

Startled back into the present. "Yes, please. Mom would you like some tea?"

"Ishbe viddle," she said.

Holly's eyes filled with the caring concern so often seen in all the Home's staff members. "Why don't you and Faith scoot up to a table and I will be right back with tea for you and your daughter, Corrine." I was at a loss for words, not understanding her gibberish. Since Holly had casually reminded her who I was, I decided to ask again. "Hi Mom, how was your day?"

Again a slur of letters that were not words came out of her mouth. She didn't appear to realize that she was speaking gibberish, and her face was unusually void of expression. Her English returned momentarily and the cause of her infrequent gibberish was never determined.

Mom was fond of company, and occasionally I brought a friend with me to spice it up a bit. I can't really tell you why, but she would be much more social and easier to converse with at times when visitors other than family members were present. It made it easier for me to have someone to converse with if there were any difficulties, and often there were.

Once, when we arrived, Mom was among a group watching a movie on the big screen TV. The aroma of fresh popped popcorn permeated the air and the speaker volume on high, with the bass turned up, felt like a real movie theater. The movie was called "Hollywood Chihuahua" and was about dogs. I introduced Mom to Polly and reminded her who Polly was. I never knew if it helped, but I tried to remind her of something familiar from the last time she saw them, or how she knew them. She usually managed to pretend she knew my guests even if she didn't and it helped them feel more comfortable. As time went on, she tried to be polite and chat with us, but was still interested in her movie, so we just watched it with her. We had some nearly normal conversation and then occasional sentences with words that didn't go together as they should, but we could still figure out what she was trying to say because it had to do with the movie. For instance, she wanted to say, "That white dog is so cute," but what came out was "that 'wood' dog is so cute." It was as if she couldn't find the right word. She used the correct first letter in the word, but was unable to find the word that she needed. Sometimes, she would get this puzzled look on her face and I was sure she knew it didn't sound right, but was confused enough to just change topics. I never knew if that was intentional or just her wandering mind. You can make yourself nuts trying to analyze this behavior but it became easier to just go with the flow and accept it.

Back to the movie: Mom always loved dogs and I can't remember a time growing up when we didn't have one. She would hug them and talk to them in her own language. They wagged and wiggled affectionately in response to her voice, loving the attention! So as she was watching this dog movie with us, while looking directly at the TV, she recited a long sentence that I had heard all of my life. "Judu be datty, litty boowoo ju you." I didn't think anything of it, but my friend Polly asked, eyebrows raised, "What language is that?" It struck me funny that this time what Mom said made sense to me, yet no one else. I got a case of the giggles, and could hardly explain it to Polly. Mom joined in. No matter the state of mind, a good laugh is good for all.

The caregivers in the Home must experience these situations patient to patient, day-to-day, but I'm not sure they could even explain or comprehend this unique doggie language that Mom had contrived, somewhere between Pig Latin and the common 'Corrineism,' lovingly defined by her family. In their patient care world, it just appeared to be the normal state of her mind.

Normal Doesn't Live Here

What was 'normal' anyway? I wasn't quite sure how to answer that question for myself or anyone else. Mom's reality and my reality were separated by confusion. One thing we had in common was confusion. The more confused she was, the harder I tried to figure it all out. It became frustrating and if I expressed my frustration, she didn't understand my 'tone.' Once she said, "Why are you looking at me like you're cross with me?" It was hard to hide my feelings; after all, she was my mother and that mother part of her brain was still fully functional. For example, if we were talking about someone's upcoming birthday and she wanted to send a card, when I returned with the card that she had just asked me to buy, she thought it was for her. "Oh, thank you for thinking of me," she'd say.

At first, it was hard to not point out that she wanted the card for someone else. For some reason, it's hard to keep your own ego out of it, especially when it's your Mom. The pattern that I started to recognize was that she began compensating for her confusion by saying things that were just generic enough to suffice under the normal circumstance. How sad it was to realize how hard she had to think about everything. And then I would wonder how much conscious contemplation there really was. With things like the card, I learned not to say, "This is the card you asked me to buy for Dennis' birthday!" Instead, I would say, "I picked up this card for Dennis birthday; would you like to sign it?"

Believe me, I wasn't always so patient. I wish had learned sooner in her illness to swallow my own pride and pretend she was right. She was Mom; of course she was right. Now I can see that, whenever possible, it is a more respectful way to cope with the illness.

Clothing and Comfort

All her life, Mom always left home with her face on and dressed to the nines. As she transitioned from leopard jackets and leather pants into those dreaded Depends and assistance with her toiletries, her style of clothing needed to be easier to manage. One of the lessons here was that it is really difficult to find stylish clothing that is manageable. Manageable clothing meant elastic waistbands, tops that buttoned up the front, and cardigan sweaters for that layered look. Occasionally, a pullover sweater as long as it had a large enough neckline to not 'mess up her hair.' In the Assisted Living Home she still needed to be able to dress herself and use the restroom unassisted. What worked best now were pajamas in two piece sets instead of the nightgowns she preferred but could trip over. Shoes that were simple to get on; Velcro was better than laces that needed to be tied and untied.

Although it sounded simple to us, it had its challenges for Mom. In the beginning, she could remember her favorites from her wardrobe and would request items specifically by type, color and description. Her wishes were accommodated as much as possible as long as it wasn't a safety issue. For instance, she still liked to wear stockings (pantyhose) and dresses, but the shoe wardrobe needed to change before anything else as her instability was changing.

She had a pair of metallic gold tennis shoes that she was very fond of and when they began to wear out, Dennis went in search of gold shoes and found some in a catalog. He bought her two pair, because she was eventually happy wearing them with anything. Those gold shoes became her signature shoe in all three care Homes. Once upon a time, she had a closet of high heeled designer shoes and boots in colors to match every outfit. Now she had three pairs of Velcro Gold sneakers. Everyone knew who Corrine was - the lady who wore the gold shoes.

When it became apparent that she would not return to her own home again, we packed up her belongings but kept the clothing accessible so that she could still make requests from her seasonal wardrobe. One time my niece, Brooke, picked her up and took her to lunch and Mom wanted to go back to the house to get a favorite blouse. Mom was very specific in regards to which closet it was in. But, Brooke knew the clothes weren't there and she couldn't take her because it was best for Mom to continue to visualize her clothes in the closet where she had left them. But since that is not where they were stored any longer, Brooke had to make up a story about not having a key to the house. It bothers her to this day that she had to lie to her Grandma. There was a real issue for all of us when we were not honest with her, even though we knew it was in her best interest.

So, the woman who had incredible taste in clothing, always wore bright colors, leopard prints, high heels, makeup and accessories such as scarves and jewelry had just been rebranded, like a retail store's signature brand change. Mom had super gorgeous long legs and a very short waist, and always had a hard time with pants because they would fit above her normal waistline. If the new low-rise pants were in fashion sooner, she would have had a closet full. She would not even consider wearing sweat pants, only leggings on occasion. Her slacks had zippers and she always wore full length nightgowns and a favorite zippered leopard bathrobe with slip on, cushioned bedroom slippers. The wardrobe change to accommodate adult diapers was like a foreign costume for her. She fidgeted and wiggled and just plain was not comfortable in her new surroundings or her new clothing.

So, Mom would just get undressed and go to bed. She wasn't tired, she just knew she didn't feel right and was more comfortable in her pajamas. It was too much change, and she kept telling me stories that somebody stole her clothes. At the time, I thought it was just her confusion, but after a while, I realized that she would open her closet and in her mind, none of those clothes hanging there were hers. Well, they definitely were not what she would have chosen, given the opportunity to go shopping! With years of retail employment and a keen eye for fashion, Mom turned heads when entering a room in any environment. Her signature style became bold and bright colors that complimented her green eyes, spring complexion, and added to her ambiance. Her confidence while making an entrance into any room under any circumstance never faltered. Whether with a cane or a walker, she still announced her arrival to the party if not by saying, "I'm here, let the party begin!" then simply with the grace of her presence.

When your loved one is in any care facility, you usually have the choice to do their laundry for them or have the staff take care of it. Either way, every item needs to have their name and room number written in it with permanent marker. Mistakes are made; clothing gets lost, in the wrong basket or borrowed by another resident.

When purchasing clothes for Mom, I also kept value in mind. After she broke her hip and moved into the Home, I decided to make an attempt to keep her in the styles she loved by shopping at second hand stores. It was a lot easier to find the bright colors she liked and I even found a thick fake leopard fur vest!

This was helpful because she went through temperature phases and usually complained of being too cold. I was so excited to bring these clothes to her, but I knew with her retail discounts over the years she never shopped at thrift stores and I worried about the bag that had Goodwill written on it. Since she had retired from Nordstrom's, I pulled a little sneaky move and put the Goodwill items in a Nordstrom's bag. Ten minutes after we opened the bag and tried the clothes on, she would forget, anyway.

When I arrived with the clothes that included the special vest, Dennis was already there with Mom in the café, so I went to her room and lay the clothes out on her bed. This was a routine that Mom did for me over the years. If she picked up something to surprise me with, I would come home and she had it laid out on my bed. I didn't know if this would occur to her or not, but it was fun for me to surprise her with my great find of clothes I knew she would love. When Dennis brought her back into the room, she said, "Oh, for heaven's sake, look what we have here," and went straight to the bed. She was interested in trying on some of the more manageable items and the rest we put in her closet.

It was a good visit that day and I can still see how cute she looked with her leopard fake fur vest on and her big beautiful (toothless) smile. She continued to wear that leopard vest, day in and day out!

One day when I arrived, Mark, my favorite nurse, said, "she's fidgeting today and I'm not sure why." She had changed her top twice and was still complaining it wasn't comfortable. When I sat with her, she kept pulling at the ribbing along the bottom of her shirt and I asked what was wrong. She said, "This just doesn't feel right," and she kept pulling it up like she wanted to take it off. It was right side out, with the tag in the back so I tried to tell her it was fine and distract her with the book I brought for her to read. She would have none of that, and kept fidgeting. We changed her top to a button up blouse and that still bothered her. The combination of Mom's short waist, sweatpants up to her bra-line and Depends was frustrating her. She repeated, "It just doesn't feel right!" I tried a few more adjustments, but still could not make her comfortable.

As she sat there in a state of frustration, pulling at her shirt again, she said, "It feels like my boobs are clear down at my waist!!"

"Well, that's because they are! And for more reasons than you want to admit!"

Mark came in and said, "You two have made my

day!"

Always Accessorize!

Accessories were a necessary part of who Mom was. Scarves, bangle bracelets, Earrings, two rings minimum on each hand. Unfortunately, it became easy to lose things that were not consistently in the same place. Purses and scarves could get left on a chair in the café, or dropped in the hall. She just loved her jewelry. There came a time, when wearing it in the assisted living facility clearly was not a good idea. She had already lost several thousands of dollars in false teeth and we didn't want her to lose her jewelry, too. The aides said she was taking it off at night and forgetting where she put it. This was around the same time as the pink punk rock hair and the green eyebrows. Dennis, concerned, decided to take her jewelry away and we all agreed it was the right thing to do. Well, everyone agreed except Mom. Talk about something of habit stuck in her head! She claimed "I wouldn't lose it, why on earth would I lose my jewelry?" She insisted that she never took it off. This reminded us of the car keys and we knew we were in for a ride.

Dennis convinced Mom that her jewelry needed to be cleaned. He took it from her and gave it to me to clean. I kid you not, for six months, she asked about her jewelry. I would watch her run her fingers across her hands and then she would ask. She was so used to feeling her hands with the jewelry, having worn it as long as I could remember. I told her things like "the jeweler went on vacation right after I dropped it off," and she remembered her favorite jeweler so I would tell her," he said to tell you hello and asked how you are doing." *Little white lie.* I would promise her that I would call and check on it. Then after some time, she told the story so many times that it took on its own evolution. She embellished it a little more each time. I was traveling overseas for business at the time and she got it in her head that I took her jewelry to London to a jeweler over there to have it cleaned. "When Faith went to London to get it," her make-believe story continued, "it was a holiday and his shop was closed." The last time she told it, the jeweler had gone out of business and I had to go to London and get it back. The strange thing is that every time she would bring up her jewelry, she would rub her hands and fingers and say she missed it. Her mind remembered the feeling of wearing the jewelry and that memory far surpassed other clothing concerns, makeup or even the teeth. This was a very curious and intriguing memory connection.

Her wedding ring, for instance, was a collection of family gems. Its history was priceless. She had received her Aunt Louise's rings, her mother's wedding ring and, with some of her own jewelry, decided to put them all into a single gold band and thus creatively display the family jewels. I remember going to Sausalito with her; a friend had told her a jeweler there could make that style of a ring for her. She had an idea of what her design would be and I remember climbing the narrow stairs up to the quaint jewelry shop while Mom laid out the stones on a tray of black velvet and explained what she envisioned to the jeweler. It was a very small shop, where he made beautiful and uniquely crafted custom jewelry. He was an elderly gentleman with a long white beard and as we left his store and walked back down the narrow stairs, Mom sounded quite concerned when she said, "I hope he doesn't lose my diamonds in his beard."

Once the ring was created, she loved it and it was her favorite. She wore it until we had to take it away from her. Once, years ago, that ring went missing and Mom was so worried, she said she felt sick to her stomach. She thought she might've dropped it while in the bathroom and thought that it could've gone down the toilet without her noticing. She convinced Dad to remove the toilet and investigate and see if possibly the ring was reachable inside the drain. Dad went diligently on this gross treasure hunt, this labor of love, without finding Mom's ring. Months later, we heard loud shriek of joy.

Mom had found her ring. Dad and I joined her in the living room where she described that she had dropped a cookie and reached between the couch cushion and the back of the couch and found the ring she had searched for so desperately.

Perfume

Mom's favorite fragrance was Ciara by Revlon. When she heard it was being discontinued, she insisted that we purchase it whenever possible. It was her signature scent. When we realized she was never coming home and we packed up the house, we found hoards of little boxes of Ciara tucked away in drawers and closets. Once she imagined it was going to be discontinued, she was determined to keep a stock of it. The nursing home discouraged the use of perfumes because, as you can just imagine and given their clientele, there is only so much aroma of 'Gardenia', 'L'aire du Temps' and 'Ciara' one cafeteria can handle in a day. And, given the overall geriatric populous and their deteriorating sense of smell, there was an overabundance of fragrant layers. I can still smell it as I am writing this.

Memory Moments Beyond 'Normal' Dementia

As you witness this progression, you get to a point where you begin to recognize the cycles of confusion. Sundowner's Syndrome is that fatigued state of confusion unique to evening. Eventually, I tried to reduce my evening visiting hours because of this and you may, too. Evenings were much more frustrating for both of us. Remember the time she didn't want to return to her room and thought she was supposed to be at work? That was an evening after my workday, which was around 7 p.m.

One Sunday when I was there with her in her room, she told me that, "those people on the freeway are driving too damn fast and I can't go anywhere! There is just too much traffic."

I didn't have a clue what she meant and asked "Who?"

"The ones out there," she replied while motioning towards the hallway. There were a couple of patients with motorized wheelchairs and I thought that she meant they were driving past her doorway a little fast. Then she asked me if I would help her with something.

"Of course," I replied, "What do you need?"

She said, "I need you to get these butterflies out of my room."

"Butterflies?" I asked.

She replied, "They are circling overhead and driving me batty!"

Well, one thing was for sure, there were not any butterflies in her room and that was not a freeway of traffic outside her door. I asked how she felt, and she told me she really didn't feel very well and wanted to lie down. So I checked in with the nurse and told him there were butterflies in her room. It was Mark, Mom's favorite male nurse. He raised his eyebrows and asked if I needed help catching them. He appreciated her good sense of humor, and I could see why, he was being a bit witty himself today. She was always very flirty with him and he was not only a good sport but a good nurse and decided to check her urine for a UTI (Urinary Tract Infection.) For whatever reason, a UTI in the elderly can cause confusion, "butterflies in my room" type of confusion. After we got her all snuggled into bed, I kissed her good bye and teased her about dreaming of butterflies as I left. Mark called me later to tell me that Mom did have a UTI and the resident physician had started her on antibiotics. It was nearly routine for him, since urinary tract infections are common amongst the elderly, once again in diapers.

I realize that I just happened to be there at the right time to experience the butterflies, and I trust that the Home would have determined this was an issue just as quickly. In this situation, she was fortunate to have very good care and a group that communicated well between shifts. This allowed her family to just stop by whenever it was convenient. Unfortunately, all nursing facilities do not have the luxury of adequate staffing, to satisfy both affordable care and quality care.

While we are on the topic of adult diapers; I found it incredibly hard to tell a loved one when it is obvious they need a diaper change. It is easy to openly state the facts with a small child, but I really struggled with announcing this to my mother. Subtle hints, such as, let's go to the bathroom before we leave, or putting a towel on the seat in the car. It is just plain awkward, and there is no easy way around it. Often, she wasn't in a cooperative mood and would deny her needs and my assistance. The skilled staff was always very helpful when an outing was planned and they can manage all those necessities in advance. Enlist the aid of the staff as needed; it is routine for both patient and staff and can be less awkward for you as well as the patient. I knew that she would want me to help her to maintain her dignity so I had to find a work-around for her independent nature in order to do so.

There were three types of memory issues beyond her normal confusion; Sundowners, UTI's and medicated confusion such as the sprinklers dancing on the ceiling. Awareness that there can be additional memory impairment will help you cope with the day to day confusion and recognize potential secondary influences.

Dancing Queen

Mom always had an incredible talent when it came to rhythm and dancing. She joined a performance group when she was 75 and performed as a tap dancer until she was 87 years old. Given her age and a very active lifestyle, she developed arthritis in her knees and was having more difficulty getting around; the doctor advised her to slow down. She laughed in her flirty Mom way and told him "I don't do slow!" He persuaded and explained that she didn't have to stop everything but she had to make a choice in order to reduce the painful inflammation. She led us to believe her choices were to either give up walking around Greenlake every day or to cease tap dancing.

Greenlake is a three mile paved walk and she drove there, met a friend and they walked together darned near every day. Although some motion and exercise is good for arthritis, she was not going to give up her love of dancing! Walking may have been easier on her knees, but dancing was good for her soul and social health. Gradually, she started losing her balance on stage and her fellow dancers were afraid she would hurt herself.

Tap dancing is a mind stopper, for sure. In order to

focus on what your feet are doing and keep time to the music, tapping at the proper moment in sync with the group at the level of required perfection, there isn't any way your mind can wander and still manage to keep in step. It is like drumming, only with your feet instead of drumsticks. I took a few classes and developed a respect for Mom's ability to not only sustain the physical competence and energy required to tap dance, but also her ability to remember all the steps in each dance. She kept it to herself as long as she could, but it was a sad day when she had to admit to herself and others that she just couldn't remember the steps anymore and was making too many mistakes. Her friends recognized how difficult this decision was for her and were wonderful in helping her through the transition. They even choreographed shorter segments of a dance to give her the recognition she adored and less to remember while on stage.

Dancing at her advanced age allowed Mom a continued life beyond retirement and she blossomed as if with a second wind. She found new friendships and a wonderful support group that extended outside dance rehearsals and performances. It made her feel young and alive again and grateful for the experiences she shared with such joy. They performed on cruise ships, nursing homes (Mom called them 'Old Folks' Homes,) the 5th Avenue Theater in Seattle, the well-known Victorian Country Christmas in Puyallup and many other locations. Mom's dance friends ranged in age from thirties to eighties and are still donating their time and efforts performing. Beyond just performing, they made their own costumes and stage sets. We have photos with, fabrics and lace, feathers and hats and glitter and glue strewn from one end of Linda's dining room table to the other.

Mom was one of the eldest in the performance group but was preceded in death by several of her very good friends. It was not uncommon to find her taking friends or their families pre-made dinners, sitting by their side if needed and openly sharing her love for life through laughter as well as sharing their tears.

After Mom had been in the Home for a while, one of her former dance partners, a good friend, passed away after an extensive battle with cancer. When Mom's friend, Linda, called to tell me the news, I agreed that Mom should know in case she would like to attend the service. But, would she remember him? Linda and I took pictures of her and Ed in their dance costumes, sure they would jog her recent memory. We were disappointed once again. When she looked at the photo, Mom just said,

"Now there is a nice looking man."

When we asked if she remembered dancing with him, the look on her face, in her eyes, frightened me. It was an expression I had not yet seen. Today, I believe that these experiences were alarming to her as well as to us. She was looking at a photo of herself beside someone she couldn't remember. But on that day, I didn't consider her feelings as we tried to entice her mind down memory lane. I was dealing with my own disappointment and it saddens me even more now to think of Corrine, trapped and frustrated inside a mind that did not work anymore. Linda told her the stories that went along with the photos and she enjoyed them as she continued to say "It doesn't ring a bell," and "I am sure he was a very nice man." She understood the loss and death, but just could not recall her relationship with Ed.

We decided that taking her to the service to see all her old friends was not in her best interest and might cause her more harm than good. Many more of her more recent memories were gone. She did seem to recognize Linda after a while, but Linda lived nearby and had come to see her on several occasions. I don't know if that made any difference or not. I also think that somehow, in some way, Mom still had enough common sense to try and not make someone feel badly if she did not remember them.

She pretended to remember. The words she chose at that point were generic enough to fit the conversation and she joked a lot. "Look who the cat dragged in" or "What brings you here today?" or "Where have you been all my life?" She avoided using names at the moment you greeted her and then she could retrieve a name after you had been there for a while. If someone asked if they were remembered when first they came to visit, they were usually disappointed. And Mom was given an added level of performance pressure when put on the spot with the retrieval of names.

Where'd She Go Now?

Mom's best friend, Madonna, stopped by on a rare Pacific Northwest sunny afternoon to find Mom taking a nap in the courtyard under a pink blossoming cherry tree. Madonna was in town for an appointment and excited to surprise her. She hugged Mom and sat down, then realized it was different now and her friend, Corinne, didn't remember her. Saddened to see the unfamiliar expression on Mom's face, she was reminded of her own mother's illness with dementia. When Madonna recounted her heartache as she shared her story with me, I regretted not knowing of her plan so I could forewarn her, perhaps meet her there. I witnessed Mom gracefully engage in conversation with many people, allowing them to believe she knew them, but she was unable to fool her best friend.

Even with dementia, habits are hard to break. The staff at the nursing home said, "She's always moving and hard to keep track of," or "She is out roaming the halls." Well, after a little analysis of her habits it all made sense to me. Mom had always worked part to full time, walked 3 – 5 miles daily, danced with her dance group including rehearsals several nights a week and always made sure dinner was on the table for Dad, even when she wasn't home. While in the nursing home, she became accustomed to using her wheelchair from dawn to dusk. The rehabilitation following her hip replacement progressed as well as could be expected, given her circumstances. When you tell a normal person not to cross their legs and they have been doing it all their life, it is hard enough to change that pattern consciously. When you tell someone with dementia anything, you need to be there to constantly remind them what you asked them to do and why. Mom's dementia got in the way of her ability to rehabilitate and walk again without assistance. The more she sat and the less she moved, the more her once beautiful and shapely legs atrophied, until she could no longer stand without shaking. She did not even have the strength to get from her wheelchair to the bed without assistance. The safest decision was to allow her to sit comfortably in her wheel chair. Some things are made easier by the dementia, particularly when the patient forgets the freedom they once had. In the prior year, if I would have even suggested to Mom she would be in a wheelchair in a nursing home, she would have had a conniption fit and told me I was nuts.

"Good afternoon, have you seen Corrine?" or, "Did you see which way Corrine went?" was now my greeting at the nurses station. Mom learned to 'ride the rail' around the hallways. There are safety handrails on each wall in all the corridors. Underneath the railings were protected corners and in high traffic areas Formica was on the lower section of the wall. Mom would grip the railing with her weathered and arthritic hands to pull the chair forward. She used her feet in a walking motion and just kept going as if she were still walking laps around Greenlake. In her mind, she had to go somewhere, anywhere, even if now it was nowhere in particular. If you asked her where she was headed, she was late for work, dance rehearsal or a hair appointment and she wouldn't even slow down long enough to talk. When she was brought back to her room for any reason - naptime, bedtime, a guest or just to use her private restroom, she would not stay long. If the nurses' aide had to leave her, the next they knew, she was back out in the hallway 'going to work.' Whatever part of the brain that retains our routines did not seem to be affected as were other areas of her memory. She had never kept still and in her mind she always had somewhere else she needed to be, although she rarely stopped in any one place for very long. They had to put the brakes on her chair when they rolled her into the lunchroom for a meal so she couldn't get away while they were trying to monitor her and encourage her food intake. Then, if it was taking them too long and she was through eating (or not eating, as the case may be,) then she let them know it!

One evening I arrived to find both Mom and Helga at the nurses' station sitting in their wheelchairs chatting, so I stood there with them. Helga always greeted me and called me 'Dear' and it felt like she remembered me. Now that I think about it, she may have come up with the generic greeting just like Mom, but it worked for me. They had already eaten dinner and were talking about nonsense. Nonsense, literally. I wondered *how do they take turns talking while not making any logical sense and still manage to appear as if they are communicating?* As I returned to their conversation, if you can really call it that, there was an announcement over the intercom about an upcoming event tomorrow. I thought, *now what is the point in that? The residents can't remember today, how will they remember tomorrow? I guess I've been hanging around here too long, I am getting a bit cynical.*

Just then, Helga began anxiously trying to roll her chair away but the brakes were set and she asked me to help her. I asked her where she was running off to, and her answer was as clear as day. "Come on, that's last call and we need to order another drink!" Before I knew it, both she and Mom were headed to the bar.

And I was worried you weren't having fun here. Who am I to judge dementia?

I Need to Get a Job!

There were times when Mom got something stuck in her head and it took weeks for it to be forgotten. Still, to this very day, I cannot understand why some topics stuck in her memory and others never even happened!

She would often complain that she didn't have any money. While at the dining table, she would ask them if they could "bring the check, please." They would tell her it was already paid for and if she asked again, they told her "Dennis already paid for your dinner." She would reply with something like, "Well, that was nice of him, and it's a good thing because I forgot my purse!" The staff took special care to know names of each resident's family members, to toss out there in conversation as needed to improve believability and it worked wonders.

In this time of many transitions, a woman who always carried a purse or a man who always had his wallet, were now without it. They didn't understand why they didn't need it, either. Just think about it; all our lives we pay for everything at the store, gas station, restaurant. It is more than just a habit, it is a fact of life. Then, they move into this nice Home that they don't really like or feel comfortable in and don't need a purse or wallet any more. Even though they don't have to pay for lunch or dinner, they don't really understand how all this is working. They each have had to earn a living and pay for anything and everything their entire life and now they don't. In most cases, they do not comprehend that their cost of living just quadrupled, and as a matter of fact, 'Mom the bookkeeper' would have had her conniption fit if she understood how much it cost for her care. It's probably best that they don't understand the price of quality care and sadly, geographically, options in some areas can be limited.

Given this new lifestyle, it took Mom a while to understand (if she ever really did,) that she didn't need to work anymore. She asked me one day if I could take her to a job interview because Rick took her car, and she didn't have a ride. *At least she didn't accuse him of stealing it this time.* I had tried to explain that she was retired, and didn't need a job so many times before that this time all I said was, "Sure, where is your interview?"

"West Seattle; it has to be close to Grandma's," she replied. *Of course it does.* This was where her mother had lived years before and in her mind, she was remembering where she lived with her own mother and needed to help support her.

Thinking about the conversation, Mom is talking to me, her daughter, as she refers to her mother as 'Grandma,' but in her state of mind, she was still living at home and needed a job. There wasn't any way to analyze this and have any logical conclusion, so I just made mental notes of situations to remember later, if needed. As if any of this superfluous data would really help me in any way. *Maybe I'm the one who's nuts*, I thought. *It all seems to make perfect sense to Mom.* Then, a few minutes later, she was back in the present and we talked about my kids, when Candace or Lauren would be home from college, where I was working, or the horses.

Another time, she told me that she needed a new job because "this one is, really boring. I work with a bunch of old people and all they ever want to do is sit around and drink coffee." And she continued to explain that she needed a job that was more interesting and kept her mind busy. Hmmm, I thought, *keep your mind busy, maybe that is what this is all about. The Home is far too boring, so she just makes stuff up to make it more interesting.* Who knows, but in every situation, I found myself analyzing why. I realize I was just trying to make some sense of it all, when you really cannot expect to find any answers. With dementia, just like life, everyone's journey is different. It is what it is, and you are where you are for a reason. "So it is," I told myself.

A call came from the Home one day. Mom had fallen. Of course, my mind immediately replayed the broken hip scenario and I was grabbing my purse ready to run out the door as they said that she had been checked out by the doctor and was fine. However, because of protocol, they needed to report all incidents to the family. She apparently had wheeled herself to the nurses' station, gone behind the no patient zone and was trying to sit at the desk so she could use the computer. When they asked her what she was doing, she insisted she had to go to work! Payroll was due and she needed that computer. During this time, she fell. When I had my janitorial business, Mom used to come over to my house and do my payroll every other Friday. It was more of an excuse to keep her active in the world of computers than to help me with payroll, but it served its purpose and was a big help. It was nice to see her on a regular basis and she enjoyed getting a paycheck, too. She had been a bookkeeper for years and could run a ten-key like no other.

Mom seemed perfectly fine when we all convened in her room that day. My witty brother, Rick, teased Mom about trying to claim that she fell at work so she could have more paid time off. Mom, on the other hand, didn't remember a thing about it.

You Never Told Me You Had Children!

As we were sitting in the courtyard one day, I told Mom about her grandson's new job. Amazed, she said, "You never told me you had children! How could you not tell me I have grandchildren?" And she was insistent and spoke with an angry tone as if she was scolding me. How do you respond to something like that? There are many ways - showing photos, replaying the past to help her remember. I had tried all that so many times, I just got to the point.

"Well you just forgot, Mom, because you used to change his diapers!" When my kids would visit their Grandma, she always knew their nicknames and joked around with them easily. But today, she didn't have any grandchildren because she wasn't old enough. I thought, *I wonder how old she thinks I am; she seems to remember that I am her daughter.*

The 93rd Birthday

It was spring break and two of my three college age children were in town. It was good timing to surprise Mom for her birthday. Sam, Lauren and I coordinated our schedules and out the door we went, cupcakes in hand, to have a little impromptu party at the nursing home. We found her in the common room, the one with a view of the courtyard. Staff service counters lined one long wall, intermixed with shelves of large print paperback books. A CD player boomed Bach's Preludio in G Major, competing with the big 60" plasma TV playing a Mariners baseball game at the far end of the room. Mom sat alone at a small table facing the courtyard, watching the birds in the magnolia tree. She was surprised when we came up from behind. Dressed in her fur vest and a sash across her chest that read, "It's my Birthday, AGAIN," she said, "Well, isn't this a nice surprise!"

We three sat with her, presented cupcakes and cards and wished her a happy birthday. She had always been such a quick wit and at the moment we didn't think anything of handing her three birthday cards and letting her open them. She still had a beautiful smile, even without her teeth, and she laughed enjoying her grandchildren. She proudly introduced them to the staff as they stopped one by one to wish her a happy birthday. She was chit-chatting with us, and read the front of the first card and then the inside, but she couldn't connect the front legend with what was on the inside. The card's humor was lost with a turn of a page.

We tried to explain the card to her, and she tried repeatedly reading the cards, inside and out, out loud and to herself, but she just was not able to understand the humor. It was probably a natural progression in her illness and state of mind, but it was a new symptom and another jolt of reality for us to experience on that day. Mom's easily-humored side, which had remained intact until now, was gone. I began to tear and couldn't let myself, for my son and daughter were laughing and loving their Grandma together, regardless.

Mom was slipping further away with each and every visit.

You Changed Channels on Me Again, Mom!

Conversations became more curious and yet, more entertaining. If I allowed myself the luxury of being entertained, they were far less frustrating. We would be in the middle of a conversation about the weather and how much rain there had been lately and what she was having for dinner and then out of the blue she would ask "And then what did he say?"

"What did who say, Mom?"

"You know, that man you were just talking to."

I thought I was talking to you. "I don't see any man, Mom."

"Well he was just standing there talking to you." she stated.

I was in the same room she was and there wasn't any man, and I wasn't talking to anyone but her. *Is it possible that she can see things I cannot see? Or is this just another make-believe in Dementia Land with Corrine?*

She would create something in her mind as if it had just happened and who knows where it came from, but the only thing that made any logical sense to me was 'changing channels.' It's like watching TV when someone else has the remote control and you are watching one show when a commercial comes on. So they switch to another show, and get interested in the next show after that commercial and all the while you are trying to figure out where this guy on the screen came from and what it has to do with what you just heard. Then you realize it's a totally different program. This changing of channels was also very common when we were driving somewhere. I'm not certain why, but I think the memory is often triggered by things we see or sounds we hear. We would be driving along talking about where we were going, and she would say something irrelevant about a blue truck. "I don't see a blue truck; what did you see?"

"The blue truck your uncle used to drive." Then she might say "I need to get back there and fix dinner for your father; you know how he has to have his dinner ready on time." Well, Dad had died three years before, but she kept acting like she just talked to him or just came home from work and fixed his dinner. If I reminded her that Dad died, she would say, "I know he died."

My sarcasm would kick in and I would ask, "Then why do you need to make him dinner?"

Her response was, "Because he asked me to." And

what do you say to that?

Sometimes I would attempt to make her understand, to bring her back to my reality. Other times, I would just run with it and see where it went. For instance, "What are you making for dinner?"

She might reply, "I think a baked potato with cheese."

Sometimes I would take it another step further, and ask "Did you already go to the store?"

Her response: "Yes, I did that this morning. I drove to QFC and locked my keys in the car and some nice man helped me get back in." *Maybe her mind needs normal, so I will try my best to give her normal.*

So I would ask, "Which car were you driving?"

She would remember and say "My car, the… (thinking hard, she couldn't remember her beloved 1989, white Buick Riviera) white one." She proceeded to tell me this whole story again, about how this nice young man helped her get in her car. I asked her where her car was parked and she described in detail where the handicap parking stalls were. It was hard to believe she made it all up because she was so convincing.

I thought, *she must have pulled this story from the archives stored somewhere in her mind.* I eventually asked her what she got at the store, but by that point in time she couldn't remember, nor did she remember she was fixing Dad dinner. And sometimes her comeback would be something that contradicted her original story, like, "Why would you think I went to the store, how would I have done that? You know I'm stuck here without a car" with an attitude questioning me like I was the one out of my mind!

I thought, *she is back to reality, for the moment.* Then she would change channels again back to something entirely different. *She thinks she needs to make Dad dinner, but she doesn't have a kitchen anymore. She says Dad is here. Maybe he is here in spirit and she can see him.* The past was comforting to her so I ignored my insecurities and accepted my new role in Corrine's stage play to allow her the freedom and comfort and did my best to follow her lead.

Life with dementia is full of reruns and channel surfing. While having one conversation, Mom would often ask a totally isolated question that did not relate to any current event, topic or present conversation. I racked my brain trying to keep up with her. She would have something stuck in her mind and keep returning to it. It could be something we just talked about and had to talk about again and again, the rerun portions of our conversations. It didn't ever seem to help if I told her, "Mom, I already told you," which was easy to do in a normal conversation with your normal mother. Managing my own personal growth while managing Mom's illness was a continual effort that stretched my patience like a pair of ill-fitting leggings.

Another time she told me she couldn't talk to me for very long because she had to go pick up a friend at the airport. When I asked who she was picking up, she couldn't remember. Then she told me she had made the trip to the airport earlier in the day and traffic was just awful! Again she was so convincing when I asked which way she went, she very accurately described I-5 in detail, where the traffic was stopped, and how long she waited, but couldn't remember its name.

I refer to this as changing channels because so many times we would flip conversations back and forth, from the past to the present. From gibberish nonsense to a lucid conversation. She would ask me "How was work?" or "Did you feed the horses yet?" Or a string of words that did not belong together. Some days it was exhausting just trying to follow where her mind went.

One day, she was gazing out the window looking past me. There was nothing out there but the trees in the courtyard so I asked her, "Where did you go, Mom?"

"On a trip," she replied. All I could do was laugh, because in her present state, that had so many meanings. It was just like her to share her quick wit at a moment when you thought she was long gone.

I arrived once when she had fallen asleep in her chair. Her Kelly green sweater was buttoned unevenly, the center bubbled in between the buttons. I quietly sat down and watched her sleep. Her gnarled hands were curled up under her chin, supporting her head. With her teeth out, her mouth was sunken and enhanced her high German cheekbones, the cheekbones she was proud to have passed on to me. She used to say, "You're lucky to have my cheekbones and not my beady green eyes." What a contrast it was between the perfectly groomed and accessorized Corrine I knew she would want to be, and a woman, without her teeth, hair without curl, no jewelry, and no bra. I waited a little bit, facing the fact that this was not going to get better, and I made the choice to leave without waking her up. I thought, *she won't ever know that I came and went while she was napping*, making an excuse for my own grief. As I drove out of the parking lot, I felt guilty, realizing that this time I changed the channel with my own fears foremost in my mind on that day. All I really wanted was my Mommy back.

Yet another time when I visited, she seemed alert and like the Mom she always was to me. "Stand up straight, put your shoulders back, and stop scowling, you'll get wrinkles," she said. As she lectured me just like I had heard all my life, I wondered what makes this day a day when she feels like Mom again, the Mom who needs to remind me how to properly present myself?

Then we went on to talk about the parakeets that we had while I was growing up. One was named Brody and one was named Brandy. Mom told the story about Brody playing on the floor in the small kitchen with the ball, tossing it to his left while she was trying to make Thanksgiving dinner without stepping on the dumb bird. Brody used to fly just above the ball so that the air from his wings would push the ball and make it roll across the floor. The kitchen floor was uneven in that old house, so the ball always rolled back towards the kitchen sink, and Mom used to kick it to the other side of the room. It was as if she was playing soccer with a parakeet and a plastic ball while she was fixing dinner. So, another day when she seemed very lucid I asked her: which bird was it, Brody or Brandy, that used to play ball with her on the kitchen floor? She looked at me with a blank stare as if I was speaking a foreign language and asked "Did you bring the ice cream?"

Ornery Mood

One day after work, I found her out roaming the halls and wanted to take her back to her room. I had brought my dinner with me and some French fries for her and thought that we could sit in the privacy of her room while we ate. I thought it was easier to share our food alone together than to eat out where I may confuse other residents by eating in front of them. First she told me she was busy and didn't want to go to her room. I coaxed her with the French fries and wheeled her all the way to her door when she decided she was NOT going in! As I turned the chair to make the right turn into her room, she put her arms outstretched and held on to the doorjamb. With feet squared to the bottom of the doorjamb, she yelled like a young child. 'No, stop, I don't want to!' *Is this happening? My 93 year old mother in her gold Velcro shoes is blocking my way through the door while at the same time throwing a temper tantrum.* I continued to tempt her with the French fries, but she would have none of it! One of the nurse's aides could see I was having a little trouble handling her chair, my dinner and drink tray and Mom's little tantrum. She came over to see if she could help. In her kind and gentle way, she reminded Mom that she loved French fries and that we needed to go into her room to eat them, and with that direction, Mom cooperated.

We were finally in her room. While handing her the French fries, she said "I don't want these. I have to go to work!" Sometimes there just were not any words to say when she was in a mood.

Tired and hungry, having worked all day, I was looking forward to sharing my dinner and catching up. She seemed fine with that, but it only lasted a few minutes before she was rolling out the door, telling me she was late for work! Too tired to fight with her, I sat there in her room in deep thought about this journey. *Where does she go when she goes to work?* As I finished my dinner, watching the news on her TV, the aide came back in and asked, "Where is Corrine?"

"She was late for work."

She laughed and said "I'll go find out what time she'll be done for you." Soon, she wheeled Mom back into the room, smiled and said, "I think she's off work now, the store is closed."

Mom didn't remember any of the aforementioned events, just smiled and said, "Well, when did you get here? I didn't see you come in." I handed her the French fries and she thanked me and we started conversing as if I had just arrived.

Another time stands out in my mind. Again, she didn't want to be in her room, although they preferred she stay there. It was their three p.m. naptime and all the residents were resting except for my stubborn Mom. The aides would let her stay in her chair and sit at the nurses' station if she insisted. It didn't really surprise me; she wasn't really one to ever take a nap unless she didn't feel well. This habit went along with the 'never stopping' mode she followed, always going from one activity to the next throughout her active life. Frequently, she would fall asleep in her chair while she sat at the nurses' station, but she was not about to lie down and take a nap because she wasn't tired! *Smile*.

On this day, I wheeled her back to her room to have a quiet conversation and she pulled out all the stops at the door again. This time, Mark was there and he came to my rescue. She was very loud while telling me, like a small child throwing yet another tantrum, "I don't want to go in my room." She even stomped her feet.

I scootched by her to get through the doorway and into the room and said again and again, "Mom, come in here with me, please." She sat out there and started scolding me, her voice loud.

Mark tried to jolly her along. "Corrine, this is a Rest Home and people are resting. I need you to keep your voice down, please."

She ignored him and stared at me through the doorway. "You come here this minute, young lady. If you don't behave, I am never bringing you back here again!" *Really? It is pretty rare for me to be without words, but I honestly don't know what just happened and where she went in her head. First, she didn't want to go in 'her room', and now she thinks she brought me here, and I am no longer an adult, I am a child, and believe me, I would rather not be here either!"* This one I had to think about for a while.

Mark came to the rescue and brought an ice cream to distract her, wheeled her into the room and kidded me. "I guess you know where you stand, young lady." One thing for sure, you have to maintain a sense of humor working with dementia patients day in and day out, and Mark had adapted lovingly.

On this day, her mood continued and she started complaining about her roommate, telling me stories about Helga going through her closet and stealing her clothes. Her roommate was lying down in her bed in the same room with only a curtain between us. I was trying to remind Mom that it wasn't polite to talk about people that way, and I tried to explain that Helga was most likely just confused and looking in the wrong closet. Her attitude was combative and I decided that I couldn't play these games today. I told her that this wasn't any fun and would come back when she was in a better mood. She whined like a child, but I made my exit. I think I was trying to convince myself that it would be better next time.

It was a blessing for Mom to have a staff with the patience and resilience to deal with her changing moods on a day to day basis. If I had carried out my plans to keep Mom at home and care for her, I could not have just walked away and said 'I'll come back later when you're in a better mood.'

The Patient Quarterly Care Reviews

I called these quarterly meetings 'Parent Teacher Conferences,' because that is what it felt like. My brothers and I had become the parents, making decisions about Mom's care. There were times when she had misbehaved and we needed to talk to her about it, about being kind to other residents, or as I called it, 'playing well with others.' Being kind was Mom's nature, but now she seemed to forget her manners at times. She was 'written up' once at the Home because she was calling one of the aides 'Fat.' She would say, "Oh, you're the fat one." Smiling all the while, she had lost the ability to understand that she was being rude.

I should explain that Mom was successful in managing her weight throughout her life, within 5 – 10 lbs of her normal weight. I don't know how she did it, but she always managed to and didn't understand why those of us that would gain and lose weight struggled so with maintaining our weight. One day I had to shut the door to her room because she started talking about the woman across the hall. Mom was talking in a very loud voice about how this woman could "barely fit in her chair she was so fat!" and as far as she was concerned, "she should take better care of herself."

These kinds of concerns became topics at the conference. We all sat around a big conference room table to talk about things that our mother needed to improve upon. The points were mostly moot, because we all knew that she wouldn't remember the conversation, but it was for the purpose of documenting and discussing the concerns. I suppose if a situation had exacerbated it was also documentation needed to substantiate a necessity for her to be expelled for misbehaving. As I left that day, I realized how vast and complex were the jobs of these administrators; seeing to a variety of concerns way beyond just quality care and the patients' health. I vowed to always honor the wonderful people who care for our loved ones when we cannot.

One time, I had been traveling a bit more than normal and although I had been to see her recently, Mom seemed to think it had been quite a while. As I entered the room, all the staff and both brothers were seated, along with my son who arrived with me. All the conversation in the room came to a dead stop when Mom looked up at me and asked at the top of her lungs, "Who are you?" My heart seemed to skip a beat. Then after a long pause, she said, "It's about time you showed up. I would like to introduce you to your brothers, Rick and Dennis." The tension lifted with our laughter, but for a brief moment, she had me. It was as if she knew exactly what she was doing!

Another time, we had been talking about her care and how much fun she was to be around and Mom said, "I have a question." The administrator, Lilly, asked her what it was. "Why am I the only one we are talking about here," Mom replied.

Lilly said, "Because you are the most important person." Mom's sweet smile was huge. Then the nurse mentioned that Mom was always keeping them on their toes, telling them what to do. Mom replied, "Then we have a big problem," the nurse acknowledged her and asked her why. Mom said, "If you need me to tell you what to do, then we are really in trouble!"

DNR

One of the most difficult decisions to make in a loved one's care is the point of no return. Upon admittance to hospitals for surgery, you are asked if you want to be resuscitated if things go wrong. Dependent upon age and medical conditions, the most common answer is 'yes, please resuscitate me.' However, there comes a time when it makes sense to sign the Do Not Resuscitate order, referred to as a DNR, which prohibits staff from resuscitating the patient in the event of the trauma of heart failure.

Given the state of the patient's dementia, you have just rounded the bend to question, is the patient capable of making this decision? In Mom's case, she and Dad both had executed Living Wills years ago, which documented the specifics of when to carry out their wishes etc. However, a DNR that had been signed at the previous facility was not in her patient file at the new facility, so they legally had to ask the question. Mom's answer was different this time. She said, "No I don't want to sign it" when they asked, which meant she decided to be resuscitated. They then had to show her exactly what it meant, as best they could.

While in the conference room with both my brothers

and me, two nurses, the social worker and the facility administrator, they brought in a Resusci-Annie and laid the aptly named mannequin on the table. One of the nurses showed Mom what had to happen should the heart stops. They explained all the details about the risk of cracking ribs and physical damage while the heart was being aggressively compressed. With all of us witnessing her decision, she said, "Yes," and signed the new form confirming that she understood the request to not be resuscitated. There was a medical power of attorney in place and we all agreed that in her right mind, her decision had been clear and well documented.

They moved Annie off the table and we continued our conference, discussing her current list of medications, the progression of her illness and any changes needed in her care plan etc. We each had to sign the form to say we were present and had all witnessed her decision and we were each offered a copy of the document. As we were clearing the table and Rick was starting to wheel Mom towards the door, Mom's mother voice commanded, "Stop! Wait a minute!" She pointed to Annie the mannequin, still lying on the floor. "Aren't you going to let her get up now?"

Good old Corrine would 'come to the party' when she realized that we were all there to talk about her and she was center stage. Center stage was always her comfort zone. Even in her confused state, she recognized that she could make everyone laugh, and she did. I would like to think that Mom's conferences were as fun for the staff as they were for us.

Whose Mind Is It, Anyway?

As we take this journey down the path into Dementia Land where everything becomes a world of make believe, we can't help but stumble. Hand in hand, we trudge the paths of a world all created and concocted within the afflicted mind. The world is their journal of trips to the store that didn't happen, and conversations that caused them to laugh out loud but didn't make any sense, and frustrations with things that we 'normies' cannot see or hear. As one of those normies, a family member, it is difficult to express how this feels to you, and impossible to know how it feels to the patient.

I repeat for emphasis: I didn't see that I was in denial as much as I was. The bottom line was, Mom was here in body, she was still full of life, but the Mom that knew all the things that mothers just know, wasn't in there anymore. There was this nice woman who couldn't remember my childhood any longer or the wonderful moments we shared during the birth of her grandchildren. She couldn't remember that I purchased her home and wanted to continue hers and Dad's wishes to keep it in the family. The Mom that always had a 'To do list' and a calendar full of places to be, now didn't know where she was or where she was going. However, I will be ever grateful that she always knew my face and smiled, appearing to recognize me when she saw me. I have friends that experienced the, "Who are you?" question and had to face an even deeper reality of emotion than I did. I can only imagine how much that hurts.

The woman who had been a walking travel magazine of details, now could no longer answer questions about our international travels and which pictures were taken in which city, and what year. When we lived in Turkey, both Mom and I learned to speak enough Turkish to survive life in a foreign country. We needed to communicate while shopping or ordering in a restaurant and over the years we continued to share that little bond of words only we could understand by greeting each other in Turkish on occasion.

In the beginning of this journey, I would greet Mom saying "*Marhaba, Nasilsiniz*" and she would reply, "*Marhaba, Nasilsiniz,*" which is simply, Hello, how are you? This lasted for many years until one day I greeted her in Turkish and she just looked at me like I was nuts, and said, "What, honey?" I said it again, and tried to remind her of the years we lived in Turkey, but she gave me a blank stare with no apparent recollection. I had to accept that I have many memories that we shared, but are now the memories are only mine because the two people with whom I shared them, Dad and Mom were, one way or another, no longer here.

A loss is a loss, even when you are looking the loved one in the eye. My grieving process began before she left. And although I wish I could spare you from experiencing that awareness, it is inevitable that you will. Loving someone and losing them is a loss to grieve and a part of living. I just didn't ever consider grieving the loss of someone while they were still staring you in the face.

<u>Mom's 94th Birthday</u>

At 94 and time to celebrate, Mom seemed like she would just keep on truckin' through each challenge as her mother had. I secured a room at the Home and invited everyone there because it was easier for her to stay where she was than to leave. She became confused when she was in a car or a new place; it was obvious that it was best to keep her in familiar surroundings. I coordinated sandwiches, cake and ice cream, plates and silverware, coffee and condiments etc. On my way, I stopped at a party supply store and got her a Birthday Crown, which may seem silly, but she still loved being the center of attention and had not a care in the world for what anyone thought of her.

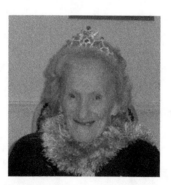

When everything was ready, I placed the crown on her head and Rick wheeled her to the conference room and surprised her with nearly the entire family.

My cousins were there and although Mom could not recall their names at first, it didn't take long before she was calling them by the childhood nicknames she had bestowed upon them as her young nieces. They were close in age and had spent lots of time with their Auntie Corrine, particularly in the summer time when school was out. They had always played a game with her, asking, 'Which one of us is your favorite?' Lynne and Priscilla joined Mom at the table and of course that topic came up. Mom fell right back into the role of Auntie Corrine, and joked around like she always had.

Mom listened while Priscilla and Lynne caught up on kids, life and their personal journeys fighting cancer. Priscilla brought up summer break, swimming in the lake and how much she enjoyed those times. Lynne remembered sitting side by side in the lawn swing with a bowl in her lap peeling apples for pies. "I still think of that to this day when I bake apple pies, Corrine." Lynne continued, "I am not sure if I ever thanked you for all the beautiful hats you knitted for the boys Auntie Corrine, so thank you."

Mom started to respond as Priscilla interrupted.

"What hats? I didn't get any hats!"

"She always liked me better, Pris!" Lynne continued. "Ok Corrine, once and for all," and Priscilla chimed in, too. "Who is your favorite niece?"

With a devilish look in her eye, Mom smirked at Lynne while pointing her finger at Priscilla. While we were recovering from the laughter, Corrine reached over to Lynne's heart necklace, pulled the chain up and said, "You should shorten this, it would look better up here." Lynne cradled her hand over Mom's while they both held the chain up and said, "I think you're right, Corrine, you still have your good eye for fashion at 94!"

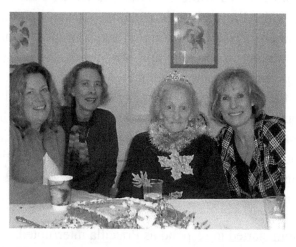

Priscilla and Mom reminisced travels and cruises

together and Lynne talked about the Husky Football games and their trip to the Hawaii Bowl game. It was a good party and gave us all a pleasant memory to hold in our hearts.

When it came time to read her birthday cards that day, she tried to read them out loud as we all listened. I heard her attempt to read the words, but gibberish was all she spoke. She had reached the point where she could not read out loud, or recognize or pronounce the words on the page. We listened carefully to her disconnected words; we could not patch them together in any logical way. I am not sure if she realized it or not, but in an effort to shield the embarrassment from her, or us, Dennis and Rick read the cards aloud to her instead. She loved reading so much and now another part of her had been taken away. With a nod, as if choreographed in agreement, none of us wanted to break down and cry during Mom's party.

What caused Mom to Arrive in This Place at This Time in Her Life?

There is much research to determine the cause of dementia and Alzheimer's and those of us who have experienced the loss of a loved one are curious and long for answers. Clinical research shows that subtle things such as exercising the brain, will help delay it. I have met people while traveling that are actively playing word games like Sudoku or working crossword puzzles, for this very reason. These do keep the brain exercising. What did not make sense to me was that Mom worked into her seventies as a bookkeeper, which takes a lot of analysis and brainwork. As did her talented hobby and love for tap dancing. She tap danced until she was eighty seven, learning new dances every week. In the process of learning the dance, rehearsing each step in the choreography, your mind must keep focused on what your feet are doing.

As far as diet and vitamin deficiencies, research indicates that potassium deficiency can contribute to memory loss. In hind sight, I do recall that Mom was potassium deficient. She used to crave bananas and eat dehydrated banana chips and baked potatoes. Listening to our body's cravings is important. The body's messages and cravings married with supporting blood work analysis, indicate that we should learn to pay attention to our cravings. Our bodies are trying to tell us something.

I wonder how much diet contributes. From a natural perspective, think about all the chemicals and unnatural products in our popular foods, and then consider the overall decline in our nation's heath. Does our diet of processed, high fat foods contribute as well? As for Mom, along with the craving for baked potatoes, she also craved the fats. I remember asking "Why don't you have a little baked potato with your margarine, Mom?" I do not have any supporting clinical research for this theory, it has just occurred to me as a possibility.

I do not know what caused my mother's dementia. Could it have been triggered by the previous head trauma, undiagnosed mini strokes, or the possible link to low estrogen levels, yet nothing substantial showed up in any of the tests to support a given cause. Sometimes I think it may have been a God moment. Counting blessings, if her memory had been intact, it would have been much more challenging for her to accept the need for care. It occurred to me that Mom did not like putting her own mother into a nursing home and was determined to live in her own home and take care of herself. However, when it became impossible to do so and Mom needed care for her physical needs, her deteriorating mind allowed her the grace to do so almost willingly.

I should note that my analysis of Mom's situation is as purely speculative as a daughter trying to make sense of it all, and is without any scientific basis.

The Slippery Slope Downhill

Life took a sudden left turn, with difficult times around every bend. The family gathered for a wonderful Mother's Day brunch at the Home. They really did a nice job making all the mothers feel very special in a more formal dining room than the standard cafeteria style setting. The tables were dressed in linen tablecloths and napkins, decorated with vases full of flowers and a bottle of champagne for mimosas. "Breakfast fit for a king," Mom said. The long side tables hosted a full on buffet with a variety of entrees, meats, potatoes and fruits. Remember, Mom's food needed to be pureed or cut and smashed so she could gum it and swallow. Dennis, Sam and I went through the buffet and chose a selection that worked for that purpose, while Rick kept her company. It had become a habit for us to just make choices for her because even if we told her what was on the menu and asked her what she wanted, by the time we returned with her plate she didn't remember what she had requested. At first this felt disrespectful, but like all other necessities, we adapted.

This day began full of joyful laughter but, part way through the meal, Mom choked on her food and several of the staff raced over to help. Within just a few seconds, we were surrounded by the staff including the nurse, and they swiftly tended to Mom and the events that evolved. What apparently happened was part of the progression of the dementia; Mom forgot how to swallow. I never thought about this being a function of a memorized muscular action because we all seemingly do it automatically. However, since all of our bodily functions are controlled by the brain, as the brain synapses fail, so can the function they control.

The beautiful table was a in a state of disarray and none of us were interested in finishing our meals. Concerned for Mom, we quickly took her back to the privacy of her room. She hadn't really eaten much, but was afraid to eat because she remembered the choking and it upset her. Odd, but because of the heightened fear of the experience, it stayed with her as it did every time she choked over the next month. She made up her mind that she would not eat anything solid. At first that seemed OK because the nutritional drinks were so well supplemented, they could sustain her for quite some time.

Everything in a nursing home is well documented. They did their best to log every meal and how much remained on the patient's plate in order to determine the nutritional intake. Since Mom adored chocolate, it was easier to get her to drink a chocolate flavored meal in a can that to eat pureed food. After the Mother's Day brunch episode, I thought all would be well because she could still drink the liquid supplements as prescribed by the doctor. A short time thereafter, the staff called to say she was also choking on the liquids as her ability to swallow was declining. In their experience, this was common and consistent with other dementia patients. The only other nutritional option to sustain Mom was a permanent feeding tube.

Mom had a Living Will, as well as the DNR. We needed to honor her Living Will. Although we all remembered it differently, when the three of us sat down and read it together with the nursing home social worker, it was crystal clear. She did not want to be on a feeding tube, IV or any type of life support at this stage of her life. Having this document was a gift; it did not place the burden of a difficult decision on the family. The toughest part was behind us as far as making a decision. I encourage you to make sure your loved one has considered these options while they are still able to make the choices. It is very common now and most hospital administrators inquire and request a copy as needed throughout the course of admission or as the need for care progresses.

It wasn't easy, of course. The documentation provided clear instructions for family and medical staff to follow. It allowed us to feel that we were doing what Mom wanted. The body does not want to starve; it wants to nourish and mend. However, I believe that Mom made a conscious or unconscious decision to stop eating. She didn't ask, or say she was hungry. While she was offered nutritional drinks and thickened liquids, she continued to politely say, "No thank you." If she was thirsty, and wanted something to drink, we provided it, but because she eventually could not even swallow water, the natural occurrence was dehydration and in a slow and natural progression her organs slowed down.

The Home's caring professionals asked if we wanted Hospice to be involved. Hospice is wonderful, especially when you bring a loved one home if they chose that as part of their care plan. We used Hospice for my dad and I cannot say enough for the caring guidance, support and wisdom shared with the family. In the very difficult time of experiencing the death of a loved one, their knowledge and experience is invaluable. In Mom's case, she had such good care with the Home, we asked them to determine if they felt the additional care and assistance would help Mom and asked them to choose. We were content with their care and were familiar with the process and in her case, felt that she was more comfortable where she was and did not need to be transferred anywhere unfamiliar.

When the decision was agreed upon, we kept her in her own routine as much as possible. If she asked to get up and into her chair, they assisted her as before. The staff was surprised that she just kept going even when she was not eating or drinking. On her own, as she physically became weaker, she chose to stay in bed. Each family member said our goodbyes in a different way. I chose to sit by her side and make it as pleasant as I could. Yes, it was not easy, but given the time again, I would not change anything.

I brought a small CD player and a box of assorted CD's. Rhythm and Blues, Jazz and some Meditation relaxation music. I also had some Christian hymns with the thought of calming and relaxing her, since she had always enjoyed singing at church. Sometimes I would sing along and see if she would sing with me. I still painted her nails because she loved the fact that her nails were so strong, lengthy and manicured. I guess that should be a reassurance that the nutritional drinks really do nourish. At least they produce strong fingernails.

Hospice authorized comfort care in case she became uncomfortable or inconsolable and the staff physician agreed. I do not think they ever needed to administer any morphine or medication for pain. Mom had an extremely high tolerance for pain. She didn't like the way Novocain with epinephrine made her heart flutter, so she had dental work, including root canals, without any pain control. If she was in pain, or uncomfortable in any way, she did not complain or let us know.

I will miss you, Mom – but I feel comfort knowing where you are going and I know that you will be happy.

I would like to share the experiences that Mom shared with me as she was nearing her time…I have always believed in the hereafter, and angels — but like many things in life, until you experience them first hand, you don't really believe they are possible until it is personal.

It wasn't hard to recognize that Mom's dementia made her confused and at times made it hard for her to verbalize what she was thinking or needed to say. However, I feel privileged to experience her joy during the last week, when she had many lucid moments that allowed real conversations where we shared her thoughts and she shared what she was experiencing that I could not see or feel. The following visions, as described by Corrine, occurred over multiple visits in the privacy of her room.

"Do you know that I am dying?"

So, she does understand what is happening, "Yes

Mom, I know."

"Will you be okay?"

Is she really lucid and this conversation is really happening? Wow, "Yes Mom, I will miss you terribly, but I will be okay."

While we were the only two living people in a room, she was looking towards the end of her bed and asked me, "Who are those three men looking at you?"

I looked over my shoulder towards the foot of her bed, "I don't know Mom, I can't see them, but I believe you can, do you recognize them?" *Amazing, she really can see spirits that I cannot. Maybe it is her brother Vean, her father and my dad?*

"No." She had a sweet smile on her face as she reached her arms up while looking above my head. In a sweet, soft voice she said, "I think they are my teachers…"

She asked me, "Who is that little girl?" again pointing towards the foot of her bed...

I asked, "Do you recognized her?" — trying hard to figure this all out I thought, *maybe she is being greeted by people that have passed, and maybe they are welcoming her to heaven...maybe this little girl is one of the stillborn babies that died before I was born...the sister I never met.*

But again she said, "No, but she is very cute..." as she reached up and waved her hand at the end of the bed with a big smile on her face. Then, as only Mom would do...She pointedly stuck out her tongue and laughed, like she was playing with this little girl only she could see.

Unconsciously, I turned my head again hoping that I could see this little girl, *who is she? I wish I could see this joyous child, allowing my dying mother to smile and laugh.* I couldn't help but laugh along with her. I felt a tear run down my cheek as I watched her gazing towards the end of the bed again, this time with her lips curved in a slight smile as she returned to her slumber.

***

Although understanding that she was nearing the end of her journey, I began to hope with each new visit that this enlightenment would continue and thought, *I hope she awakes again so I can see her beautiful smile, just one more time.*

As she gazed over my shoulder, I asked her, "What do you see?" I thought, *I wonder if her mother, brother or sister are here to greet her.* "Can you see Grandma or Vean or Erdean?"

She said, "Grandma was here, but she left."

Wow, there really is a spiritual presence and I am blessed to be here … I wonder if she can see the tunnel of white light we hear about … I asked her, "Can you see a light?"

She said softly, "There is a candle burning."

"Is it white?" I asked with mixed emotions, *this is true … so cool!*

She smiled and said "Yes, it's pretty." Then she put her hand to her chest and said, "When you look at it, you feel it in your heart and it makes you happy. I want to cry when I look at it."

The most amazing part is not only the spiritual experiences, but the fact that she was able to tell me, because in between these experiences she returned to her confused weakened state without the strength or words to express herself, and what she did say was incoherent.

BJ, Lynne and I met at the Home on a warm Friday evening, June 11th 2010. I waited in the parking lot so we could walk in together. They were both shocked by how thin Mom was in the short amount of time since they were last there. We knew the time was near as we each held her hands and comforted her.

This very last night, Mom did not speak. She touched us, held our hands and knew we were there, but seldom opened her eyes. I watched her raise her arms like she was reaching for something with her eyes closed and sleeping…and then as she would start to open her eyes, her arms would drop down to her sides. She did this several times and would smile softly as she reached up. She was happy to see her welcoming committee and I envisioned her recognizing loved ones who greeted her.

It was difficult to leave, but we each said our goodbyes and kissed her good night. Relieved that she was not in pain, we left her resting peacefully, comforted that she could see across the veil between our earth as we know it and the heavens we cannot yet see.

Five hours later, when the phone rang at 3:20 AM, my heart sank and I knew before I answered that Mom was gone. "Your mom is at peace now," they said.

I followed my instructions and immediately called Rick and Dennis and then sat at the dining room table, Mom's table, staring at the list of names I would call at daybreak. I made coffee and waited. Feeling both sad and anxious, I played over and over in my head what I would say when I called.

Rick, Dennis and I met at the Home to pick up Mom's belongings. While packing her room, I invited them over to Mom's house to toast our mother in her favorite spot, the one with the view of Mount Rainier. Siblings will be siblings no matter the circumstance. Dennis wanted to know what kind of beer I had. I had no idea. Sam had some Corona, and there were a few assorted stray bottles that friends had left behind. After a sibling debate about which beer was best, all the time sorting through Mom's things, I suggested Dennis just stop at the store on the way to the house and buy some beer.

Nearly every day, Mom walked out on the dock to see "My Mountain," she called it. She had met Dad the day she broke her leg skiing on Mount Rainier with a group of friends. He helped carry her down the mountain and that was the beginning. This was the end.

The gorgeous day was surely a tribute to Corrine. The lake was calm, the sun warm on our backs and the view of Mom's mountain was crystal clear. Each with our select beer of choice in hand, we reminisced, we cried, we toasted and cheered our mother's long and joyful life.

Mom had a good life and each of us holds independent memories of our personal relationship with her, and as individuals, we each deal with our emotions differently. Some have a difficult time saying good-bye or watching someone pass, some do not. No one way is right or wrong. I cannot tell you why I chose to sit by her side. It just felt to me like that is what I needed to do for myself as much as her.

There was a time in my life when death was something I feared and found reasons to avoid being present. When it was my father and mother, all that changed. I am not sure if that was because of the relationship or that by that stage of my life I had experienced many deaths and had come to terms with death or an acceptance of it. I can tell you that I no longer fear death as I once did. I cannot explain why. It may be faith, it may be learning that it just is what it is, and when death happens, you accept it in order to survive. Through each experience, I learned a little more about the process as well as learning a little more about myself.

We each come from a different place religiously or spiritually, but the bottom line is: we all deal with death in our own way and as long as we accept it there can be no wrong way. I found my mother's death to be a very spiritual experience and felt privileged to be part of it.

I hope that however your story ends, you can acknowledge that you have the ability to make your own choices along the way and that what you choose may not be what another may choose, but is what you need to do. Accept that each of us is at different places in our own journey, and what some can handle others may not be ready for. Through my experience, I now believe that your loved one who passes feels more love for you at this point in the journey than you can ever imagine. There is no doubt in my mind that they forgive you, so forgive yourself with their love.

Considering the state of their mind, or level of consciousness, you may not feel like you are able to express your true feelings because they cannot hear or understand you. Hearing is the last of the five senses to go, so keep talking! If you can allow yourself to comprehend that what the confused mind may not be cognizant or capable of, the spiritual side of the soul is ever-present and listening until we take our very last breath.

I believe that you can still clear the air by telling them how you feel, to get it off your chest if needed. It is part of the journey. The journey will continue without intermission, but you can still tell them you love them, you are sorry you crashed the car when you were a teenager or whatever else you feel you need to say. Every journey is different and every end is unique. We are here to experience all aspects of life and part of life is death. Yes, it sucks, it can totally suck, but it is still a part of who we are. Yet, you wake up the next day and grieve again, even if you thought you grieved before. No matter what your father told you as a child, man or woman now, it is healthy to cry. Let it out! It happens for a reason and it's a cleansing feeling to release those tears. Don't allow yourself to keep it in. If you do not feel comfortable crying in front of others, cry in the bathtub or the shower, or the car. Writing this book is another part of the grieving process for me. It's a good thing you are not reading the original manuscript as its pages ripple from the tears shed in its creation.

When you are in the middle of grief, you will feel like others don't understand or care and this is often true. They are in their own place; maybe they are trying to help by telling you about their day, but they just don't know what to say. You may not want to be alone with your own thoughts because they hurt, yet being with someone else can be just as frustrating because you cannot focus.

It is OK not to focus; your heart needs you to listen and to let it care. Your mind is telling your heart 'Stop, now is not a good time' or 'not now, I'm trying to work.' If you feel you are suppressing your grief, then do something about it. If you hear yourself saying, "I'm fine" — you probably are not. Here I am, way beyond death and I thought I did a pretty good job grieving both through the process and at Mom's death bed; focusing on the service arrangements helped. Yet, here I sit at the keyboard, crying with each heart wrenching story I share or laughing as I recall the joyful experiences.

I believe we are never really done grieving until we die ourselves. A memory of a loved one is the whole purpose of loving them, isn't it? So, yeah, just deal with it; it's real, it's life and emotion and it is OK to feel.

Is Dementia a Form of Divine Intervention?

In retrospect, it seems that dementia helped my Mom cope with this phase of her life with the grace and glamour that she would have wished for, given the choice. At age 90, she had lost many good friends who shared joy and happiness in her life. Dad died 10 days before Mom's 90th birthday, and after my dad was gone, if she had been left to her natural mental state, she would have been saddened by not having her friends or being able to do what she loved. If she had been aware of her surroundings, literally locked in a care facility when she had vocalized fear of being left in some Home, she might have become deeply depressed in those last years of her life. In a way, her dementia allowed her the joy of meeting new friends and sharing her love of life with them. She was still the same socialite, always smiling and cracking jokes with staff and the other residents. Even though we were saddened that she was not the same old Mom we knew and loved, dementia gave her an interesting way of still enjoying each day and sharing her joy. In the end, it allowed Mom to hide from what could have been a depressed reality of her love for life coming to an end.

Another curiosity that I share with a friend in a similar situation is: are some of the experiences we classify as dementia in our loved one really something they were able to see? Spiritually, we become aware of our inevitable passing before we, as humans, become aware of our destiny. When Mom told me she had to make dinner for Dad, I assumed she was imagining it. What if she really could see Dad's spirit hanging around her, protecting her and watching over her? She might have been confused by thinking she needed to care for him and fix his dinner, but it gave her a purpose. It was easier than when she asked me, "Where is your father? He hasn't been home for dinner in days!" The latter presented worry and concern that had no answer, whereas when she needed to fix dinner, she had a purpose and something to do that was familiar to her and by the time she got to wherever she was going, she had forgotten and was content, rather than worried.

When she thought Dad was with her, it was comforting to her. If we believe in something that isn't real, and it comforts us in the present circumstances, what is wrong with that? It's a state of mind that is our own, and really no one else's concern. I share this because I wonder if I could have had a positive effect on Mom's experience if I had understood that her imaginary visits from Dad and her mother were comforting to her. Instead, I tried to explain that they had died. The reality was painful and caused her concern and worry as to how she could have forgotten such an important memory. I forced her mind back to a sad state rather than let her exist in the euphoria that they were both still a part of her life and loved and cared for her.

Out of respect for spirituality, I now understand that it was I who could not see what was in Mom's best interest. I was stuck in my own reality. My words at this time would be, if it makes her happy, let her experience that joy and happiness. Ask her what she is making for dinner, ask her what time she needs me to pick Grandma up and where - let her believe in what she believes. It mattered not what I could not see or comprehend.

Mom really saw Dad and Grandma, but the rest of us could not. Perhaps they presented themselves to her as a comfort. Spirits may surround us, guarding us, guiding us and if we are able to see them, it is a very special gift. I do not know how else to explain it. If you can see a rainbow but it is only a vision not a defined measurable vision, does it mean it didn't happen? You didn't really see a rainbow, you imagined it? Of course not. So, I choose to believe that Mom did have frequent visits from Dad. I also believe the same with Grandma, her mother, familiar comfort to her when she felt like she was all alone in a strange place.

While Mom was a passenger in my car, she would occupy her time reading all the signs along the roadside. Business names, street names, billboards, anything with words. While reading signs out loud in the car on one occasion, something must have triggered a memory and she said, "I have not seen Grandma in a while, I need to go see her." I am grateful that I managed to say, "OK, Mom, we'll do that another time."

At an appointment with her wonderful, kind doctor who had treated Mom for a very long time, Dennis was trying to explain to the doctor about Mom's seeing Dad, and that she thinks she has to fix him dinner. As Dennis was describing her dementia symptoms, Mom interrupted him and said, 'What are you talking about? Your dad is dead, you know!" There you have it, gone from a confused woman to a lucid mother in the blink of an eye. Then a little while later, Mom looked at the doctor and said, "I think you are flirting with me; I'm a widow, you know." The doctor couldn't help but smile and give a cute reply. He confirmed that this type of confusion following the death of a spouse was very common among the elderly.

If visions are a gift of the spirit, then who are we to judge that gift? Mom saw angels at her deathbed and it was an amazing experience for me to share with her. If I had not believed that the transition from life to death could be a heavenly experience, I may have doubted her visions and chalked it up to her dementia or hallucinations. However, I am grateful that I had the peace of mind and grace to understand that what she was experiencing was a graceful passing and I am blessed to have been a part of her experience.

How Deep is the Puddle?

My emotions are at times like a puddle. I can never tell if I am just glancing at the surface or if there is something deeper there. Throughout this time, as anyone would, I was dealing with my own fears again, unrecognized at the time. Sometimes I moved through it and saw Mom even though I was afraid of what I would find when I arrived. It was as though some days I was stronger and more invincible, or just preoccupied with life and going through the motions. Other times, I left work as I had planned, drove all the way there and sat in the parking lot with an overwhelming fear of which Mom I would share time with today.

What was I afraid of, you ask? The unknown, the hurt, the panic, the pain. If I didn't like what I saw or heard, then I would have to deal with it. If we could have a normal conversation, it felt like I had a successful visit. Yet, as expected, sometimes they were not pleasant. Sometimes it was just a silly little thing that made it uncomfortable, such as her wearing someone else's clothes because hers were soiled and she didn't look like my Mom. She always seemed happy to have guests and most of the time wanted the company. I remember one particular time when I sat in the car for the longest time, talking to a friend on the phone. I should have just excused myself and gone inside; because after all, that was why I was there, right? But I think I subconsciously used the phone call to delay the inevitable, as if I was allowing my fears to sabotage the trip. The logical side of me, said, you drove here, now go in!

I have no idea what frightened me most. Possibly the thought of her not recognizing me or throwing another one of her tantrums that she didn't want me to leave her there, she wanted to go with me and she promised to be good. Whatever the reason, most of the time, I fought through it and went in. The only time I remember leaving without spending time with her was when she was asleep with her sweater buttoned up wrong. It was sometimes my schedule, but more often my emotions that determined how long I stayed. If I felt like I was going to cry, I tried to head out to the car as quickly as possible and decompress a bit. The staff was always kindhearted and could tell if I was trying to hold back tears as I passed by the nurses' station. They knew when it was time to chit-chat and when it was time to just wave, with genuine care and concern. I think I had the hardest time when Mom was in the secured floor and I needed a code just to get to her. The secure floor felt claustrophobic to me and I knew that she must feel that way, too. As time passed, the delays in the parking lot became shorter. So, I guess it was sometimes easier to walk around the puddle and get to the other side, and sometimes I needed to wade through the puddle, with Mom, each step of the way.

It is a given that you, too, will have puddles along your journey. Know that you have a choice and with that choice sometimes you need to help your loved one get through it, even when it hurts a little. Just put your boots on and march right through the puddles. You will feel better when you have done it a few times.

The Memorial Service

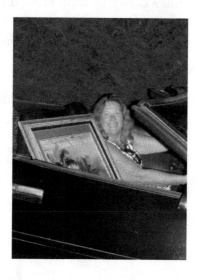

We all gathered at the church on a hot Seattle summer day in July. I borrowed a friend's Corvette and with the top down, riding in style, made the grand entrance in her honor. With the wind blowing in my hair, Mom's box of ashes, a beautifully hand-blown glass urn and oversized dance photo proudly perched in the passenger seat, I pulled the Corvette up, revved the engine and parked smack dab in front of the church steps. We were greeted by family and friends, at the same entrance I had used from preschool throughout my youth and my own wedding. On that day we said farewell to Corrine in a cheerful celebration of life ceremony.

The pastor shared our bedside conversations blessed by the angels at the foot of her bed, along with my eulogy.

I will miss you, Mom – but I know where you are and I know that you are happy.

I have always believed in the hereafter, and angels … But like many things in life, until you experience them first hand, you don't really believe they are possible. Our loving bedside experience will last a lifetime.

I hope sharing these stories helps each of you in some way, touching on that hope that we each have on our own pathway, weaving thru life's joys and challenges, while knowing all that we experience has a purpose and like a ripple on the water, we each touch and affect others' lives as we walk through our journey. I encourage you to find joy in all you do, as Corrine did, and touch many people as she did, too. I also believe that she would want you to live life, laugh loudly and love those around you — and always dance when you feel the beat.

My Recommendations To You and Your Family

Interact with your loved one often enough to see the signs. Now that you know what signs to watch for, my hope is that it just might help. Medicine is progressing at all times and the continued research in the field of memory care will surely find new treatments that are beneficial to memory retention.

Taking the following steps are difficult ones, but my experience is: it is easier to cover these bases when their mind is intact and you can make it clear you are not trying to say good-bye, but just want everything to be in order for Mom should something happen to you, or Dad, vice versa. Our expiration is one of the most difficult things to discuss with a stable mind; your goal is to understand what they want should the need arise.

Help to manage bank accounts so you not only know what banks their accounts are in, but can be alerted when there may be a risk of scams or excessive donations. This can be as simple as helping with the tax return so you can have a peek at their overall financial picture.

Know what medications they are allergic to, or food allergies. You will be expected to have these answers in an emergency.

Know what medications they take and why. Make a list. If they will let you, attend a doctor's appointment to introduce yourself; this would be a wise step and helpful later on.

Medications should be monitored, particularly if they have more than one physician. They could be cross-medicating without knowing it. If they use the same pharmacy, the pharmacist can help provide some protection, but many times these are easily missed and reactions between medications are common and can cause serious side effects.

It is wise to seek the advice of an Estate Planner, Professional Financial Planner or Investment Accountant and Lawyer that can help you determine when a Family Trust is advisable. Or find a team to cover all of the above. Many times, when planning for long term care, this option can help preserve the necessary assets. With progressive medicine, we all live longer than we used to and assets need to be protected in order to assure long term quality care as needed.

Suggest a Living Will while their mind is capable of making those logical and important life choices. The will should define if they want to be on life support or not. This includes what exactly life support means to them. Example: Oxygen to make breathing easier and a feeding tube for nutrients. Oxygen can be considered a comfort measure versus life sustaining like a feeding tube would be. There can be gray areas to discuss in order to make sure the Living Will clearly defines what they want. We all should have a Living Will in place.

If the Living Will clearly includes and defines the parameters for a DNR, then a single document may be sufficient. If not, you need to ask those questions or have the help of a medical professional to document a DNR (Do Not Resuscitate) order. These are legal documents and requirements vary by state or country, please confirm the requirements with an attorney.

Find out the burial details and preferences. It is an awkward conversation to have, but it is far better than not knowing if they already have a plot or not, or if they prefer cremation.

It's hard to put aside any prior relationship challenges when you have now stepped into the shoes of the adult in the relationship. It is challenging for the parent to allow their children to now act as their parents — both psychologically and emotionally. There are counselors who can assist with these transitions; they can mediate if a topic is too challenging to discuss. It's also a very emotional place to put yourself. It is not easy, and it can be just as difficult regardless of whether or not you have a good relationship with your parent at the time.

Be kind and caring. Try to imagine how it feels to have your privacy, power and independence intruded upon. They are young at heart and just like we avoid seeing those added pounds along our waistline, they avoid seeing themselves as old. Mom once said, "I don't know why you have me in here with all these old people, I don't have a thing in common with them. They all bore me to tears!" She was among the ten oldest people in the facility of 238 residents!

The Storage Unit

Just when I thought I was done grieving:

Sixteen months had elapsed since Mom passed. During that time, my beloved brother, Dennis, lost his battle with cancer. He was the primary estate manager for Mom and Dad's Trust. He managed to take care of most of the details while receiving chemo treatments for a very aggressive colon cancer. Although the majority of the estate details were nearly complete, there were still a few loose ends.

When Mom first moved into her memory care facility, she was allowed and encouraged to use her own furnishings and at that time, she frequently requested specific items or clothing. Dennis and Rick moved her belongings into a storage unit so that we could easily access them as needed. So now, since that was well over six years ago, I felt it was time to deal with it. I had put off the project longer and longer because I just didn't know if I was emotionally ready. The time had come to just dive into the boxes as well as the grief.

Dennis left a key for me and we had talked about where things were and what needed to be done.

When I slid open the garage door, a wash of memories combined with overwhelming dread came over me. There was the fact that Mom and Dad's life was creatively jam-packed into the 12 by 12 unit, piled upon a flood of recognition to items each having their own significance. I had seen photographs of the storage unit; Dennis had had emailed them to family along with earlier photos of the collections of furniture and knick knacks as they were displayed in Mom & Dad's house.

I was prepared to pull out things that were specifically requested by family and go to the local donation center with the rest. It was a "sight for sore eyes," as Mom would say. Staring back at me were three large wardrobe boxes stacked in the corner behind a pair of love seats sandwiched together, nested tightly with a chest of drawers holding them in place. Two to three bookcases and six dressers, a hand carved trunk supporting a TV with a stack of blankets and a porta-potty perched on top, ready to topple over. Dad's Little Rascal and walker to my left and boxes of all sizes in every nook and cranny. Pulling out two folding chairs, I sat down and surveyed the task. Dennis's widow, Donna, joined me and we pulled apart the puzzle, one piece at a time.

The memories burst out with the fragrance of Ciara lingering in the air, as I opened each box. It was as if Mom stood beside me, peering into the box, to see each and every treasure. I could almost hear her voice. "Open that one over there."

As the day went on, the sorting became a little easier. I had planned ahead and scheduled family and a friend for a short time each day, just so I didn't need to be alone with all these memories. It helped.

Tons of photos were in the unit, many of which I had never seen, pictures of trips and travels with friends, with hand written notes on the envelopes. As a result of surviving the Great Depression, both Mom and Dad saved a lot of stuff. We had already cleaned out some of it when we moved them out of the house, and I believed this storage was at least partially pre-sorted.

I found such a mixture of items packed together. Some very important old family photos mixed with a bundle of old Christmas cards. On the back of a copy of some church program were penciled notes of our genealogy. Grandpa so and so married on a specific date to Grandma so and so. If I had not turned that program over, I may have missed its significance. You see, not only does this process take time and concerted effort, one dares not omit a single step. I could have opened that box and thought, *oh, just old Christmas cards* and tossed them aside. So, step by step, I managed to pull out boxes of books and clothes that could be sorted at home. Then, I could decide if donation or resale was the best option. I found a large unframed, professionally taken photograph of my Mom when she was sweet sixteen. It is the very first time that I could see the resemblances between myself and Mom as well as my own daughters. I do not remember ever seeing this photo before, and felt the treasures stored within these walls rewarded me, one discovery after another.

In addition to the usual photos and memorabilia, I found travel itineraries and cruise ship prices, Mom's seventy year high school reunion program and my second grade report card. Notes in Dad' s familiar handwriting calculated in a little black book at what age he could retire from Ma Bell and what his pension would be. Included in this little black book were hand drawn schematics of how the multiple local telephone exchanges were wired and connected. Mom had saved assorted memories — obituary notices, memorial programs, knitting patterns, grandma's pretty patterned handkerchiefs, little butter dishes, numerous VCR tapes that were infomercials, (obviously the result of more scammed money) and candles. In the middle of the candle box was Dad's

22 pistol and its ammunition. Since we all helped pack these boxes at the house and they were packed according to location, I concluded that the pistol must have been kept in the drawer with the candles.

Dad's Little Rascal motor scooter still had the key with his aged leather wallet style keychain in the ignition. My memories ignited when I saw Dad's keychain. In better days it used to hold a boat key and car keys but now it only had his scooter key and the key to the front door of the house.

Aren't our emotions odd at times? I was also opening boxes of my Grandmother's things and they still smelled like Grandma and Mom's all smelled like Corrine. It made me wonder what my own fragrance might be in lingering wisps of memories for my children. Apparently, our sense of smell has a memory, as I didn't even have to look at the contents to recognize if they were Mom's or Grandma's.

The questions we ask ourselves are multifaceted: What did they keep this for? And then you see a little note taped to the back naming who gave it to them and it was someone special to them, so do I discard it or see if someone else wants it? Then you find something that you gave them, with a little note that breaks your heart. I had no idea that each birthday card or Mother's Day card I had given her went into a little dresser drawer. What for? Did she look at them again and again, reliving the day and my love? Given the evidence in hand, I chose to believe it was all about love, and that makes me happy.

Stuffed in a file box of papers, I found the receipt and appraisals for Mom's jewelry. Visions of her gnarled hands rubbing across each finger while she asked me for her rings, crept into my thoughts. Among the many items that I inherited, there was Mom's collection of unique jewelry from all of her travels. As I wear her favorite ring on my hand and remembered the stories, it holds a significance that makes it even more precious to me.

I found photo albums and dance programs all displayed with captions like "Corrine at the Fifth Avenue." One of them even had a pink feather used as a bookmark. The pink feather must have come off the costume with all the plumes in her hat, I thought as I looked at the oversized framed photograph of Mom in her seventies wearing fishnet stockings on those gorgeous legs, perfectly posed for the photographer. The picture had hung on the wall behind the turquoise couch at the Home. One of the staff had asked, "Why did you stop dancing, Corrine?"

"I couldn't remember the dance."

I interrupted. "Mom, you told me it was your arthritis!"

"I lied," was her simple answer.

There was also a photo of her sitting in a horse-drawn carriage, with some other dancers wearing that same costume I saw on the cover of the Victorian Country Christmas program. While reading through the program, I heard her voice in my head: "5, 6, 7, 8, brush brush, tap, brush brush tap." I envisioned my shiny patent leather tap shoes on the gold linoleum floor, trying to match the rhythm and cadence in her voice.

The woman responsible for befriending Mom and getting her involved in dancing at her late stage in life was Lynda Pressey. Lynda has this amazing energy that is contagious to all around her. I never thought it possible that Mom would forget these past years of wonderful experiences, because she had blossomed with the joy and excitement of it all. As I sat pulling memories out of musty boxes, I questioned again how all of this could be over. Just over. No more dance performances for my daughters and I to get all dressed up and attend, filled with pride watching their amazing grandmother perform with such grace and rhythm. It was just over and that was that.

One of the large wardrobe boxes had dresses and coats on hangers. I pulled them out, one by one. They inspired many memories, but one really made me smile. Lynne had told me of a time they went to the Washington Huskies football game, as she and Jim always invited Mom to the home games. The Husky colors are purple and gold and Lynne was wearing a gold lame' coat. Mom looked at her and said, "I want that coat!" Well, Lynne obligingly gave it to her favorite Auntie. And now here it was, still golden and redolent of Ciara, and I knew I had to return it to Lynne. (When I surprised Lynne with it, still another flood of memories unveiled itself. We recounted stories of Mom's excitement, sitting in the press booth with the other coaches' wives and adoring the special treatment while wearing her signature gold coat.)

As I opened the beautifully carved hope chest that Mom had used as a small coffee table at the assisted living home, I found more recent memories. I saw the skein of yarn that Lynne and I brought to Mom to see if she could remember how to knit. At the time, I was puzzled with how the mind works, and I thought about things that we remember that are functional memories like playing a piano, typing or knitting. Lynne and I planned this in order to test this theory. Looking back, I think it was to satisfy our own curiosity more than anything else. Lynne brought some cotton yarn and a pair of circular knitting needles with her and when we walked in, she handed it to Mom and said, "Hi Auntie Corrine, I need you to show me how to knit." We continued to settle in while Mom looked at the yarn and knitting needles in her hands. Then Lynne asked her if she could show her how to do a garter stitch, and Mom's immediate response was "I don't know if I can." She knew what a garter stitch was, but could not think of how to do it, so we encouraged her to try. Lynne cast on several stitches on the needles for Mom and started the first row. It took some encouragement as Mom couldn't think of how to knit in her mind, yet when her gnarled, arthritic hands started to knit, she was able to knit several stitches. Lynne and I were excited, left the knitting with her and suggested she knit some dishcloths. Since she was so focused on getting a job at this stage, we told her we could sell them and she could make some money.

Underneath the yarn were several postcards I had sent while traveling for business, telling her where I was and when I would be back. Although the cards were from a variety of places, they all reminded her that I loved her and missed her. As I read the postcards, I thought, *I missed you while I was away, I missed you while you were here and I miss you still and you are really gone for good.* But then, as I hold my own memories in my heart, I realize that she will never really be gone; she is just not here.

As life is always to be continued, there is never really, "THE END"

REMEMBER ME

Gloria Merickel, 90 - Wadena, MN

***

Dort Weeks - Holly

***

Venna Rasmussen Page, 75 - Deweyville
Mom was undoubtedly the most respected honored
member of our family. Her strength, love and
compassion kept us together during the holidays,
family challenges, and throughout her life. We miss
you mom!

***

Peggy Lambert, 67 - Edmonds
She loved her family, gardening and holidays when
she could have her kids and grandkids all together.
Even at the end, she would light up when I walked
into the room, even though she didn't know who I
was. She did on some level, know I was someone
special to her.

Doris Gregson, 83 - Greensboro
She loved her home on Rankin Mill Rd near Frank's Grocery.

***

Marilyn Wilson, 70
Mom, you always took care of everyone! You are an amazing Mom and Gram and we will remember you forever! Rest well in Heaven!

***

Albert Malgarin , 81 - Kent
Dad had a big heart and loved his family unconditionally. He shared his love with all of us through a well planned will, ensuring each of received a piece of his estate. We miss you Dad!

***

Phillis Cranney, 68 - Bothell
A wonderful mom who cherished her children!

***

Irene Baron, 60 - Minneapolis
Gone to SOON! Even to this day, all my friends still rave about your baking Mom! We all miss you!

Helen Green, 84 - Snohomish
Grammy loved us all unconditionally.

***

Naomi Duffield, 88 - Bothell
She was a friend to all with a gentle disposition. As a friend described her, "She was a FOREVER friend."

***

Janie Jones, 77 - Petal
Mom always loved telling me about the day I was born. With double pneumonia and a broken rib, the doctors did not expect her to live. After one look at her new baby girl with black curly hair and prominent dimples she decided she wasn't going anywhere! She knew in her heart I was an angel from heaven. Mom forgot this memory long ago. So now I tell HER the story of that day.

***

Sara Winters, 88 - Edmonds

***

Ruth Elian, 80 - Ft Lauderdale, FL

Maria Conlon, 65 - Washington, MI

My mom, Maria, worked in the writing world all her life from newspaper spots to human resource positions. She loved the written word and smell of fresh printed books being cracked open. She was always correcting and rewriting politicians speeches to prove she could write better ones. Her love of writing and reading will always be remembered. She still writes on pieces of paper each day … almost like she herself is writing a novel, but in a language only she can understand.

***

Olga Philips Smith, 71 - Mississauga, Ontario, Canada

Olga was a feisty vibrant mother, nana, wife, sister as well as an aspiring author who wrote a beautiful heart wrenching short story of her experience giving birth to a child with Down syndrome in the 60's. She is missed every day by her family.

***

To light a candle for your loved one, you can submit their information here:

www.journeytodementialand.com

Documents

Here are the documents that you may want to take care of ahead of time. You can find examples online. I have included Mom's NeuroPsych Evaluation for you.

*Durable Power of Attorney for Health Care

*NeuroPsych Eval Example

*DNR

*Living Will

*Last Will

*Trust

*Burial or Crematory Wishes

An Invitation from Faith

If Mom's story inspired fond memories of your journey to Dementia Land, Please accept my invitation to tell your loved one's story.

Go to www.faithmarshall.com/staying-connected for information and download the application to have your loved one's story published with our Alzheimer's and Dementia storybook. A portion of the proceeds will be shared with Alzheimer's Org programs and Awakening from Alzheimer's programs.

NeuroPsych Eval Example

One of many throughout Mom's journey.

September 18, 2003

NEUROPSYCHOLOGICAL EVALUATION

REASON FOR REFERRAL

Mrs. Corrine Marshall is an 87-year-old right-handed, married, high school graduate with consultation requested by her primary care physician, *Anonymous*, MD, to assess declining memory function in light of abnormal SPECT scan.

HISTORY

The reader is referred to *Dr. Anonymous* notes dated July 19, 2002, and more recently, this past summer, July 18, 2003. In 2002, the patient was noted to have some decline in memory and attention, and it was suspected that there may be some incipient dementia. In her review on the 8th of July 2003, accompanied by her daughter, concerns were raised that friends as well as the family have been noting memory difficulties, particularly worse in the last 4 to 6 months. There have been no significant changes in any of her medications. She scored in the low 20s on a Mini-Mental Status Exam with difficulty with some orientation, recall of only 1 out of 3 items at 2 minutes, and inability to perform serial 7s.

Mrs. Marshall then proceeded to a brain SPECT scan dated August 13, 2003. There was a large area of decreased perfusion in the left posterior frontal lobe, with smaller areas of decreased perfusion in the right thalamus and inferior right frontal lobe. It was not believed that this pattern was typical for Alzheimer disease, and the large defect in the left posterior frontal lobe was suggestive of possible ischemic etiology.

The patient is, therefore, proceeding on to neuropsychological evaluation as well as a head CT scan today. The patient's current medications include Prilosec, Vasotec, Premarin, and Paxil 20 mg.

Mrs. Marshall is accompanied by her daughter, Faith for today's evaluation, though they are separately interviewed. According to Mrs. Marshall, she is particularly noting difficulty with word-finding ability and some transient confusion when driving locally in her community, although she will not drive distances. She states that family members have noted more memory difficulties than she has. She states that she is not having any trouble forgetting to turn the oven burners off thus far and takes care of both her and her husband's medications. Her oldest son, Dennis, who has power of attorney, has taken over handling most of the checking account.

As noted in Dr. *Anonymous* notes, she has been under a significant amount of psychosocial stress with her husband who has suffered a number of falls, developed subdural hematomas, underwent subsequent surgery and rehabilitation, and was living in a nursing home until this last Christmas when he returned to live with the patient due to lack of funds to support his continued stay in the skilled facility. She denies that he has been physically abusive to her and states that she is safe but continues to be quite critical. She acknowledges that she resents having to take care of him and having to devote all of her time to him. She thinks that the Paxil has been helpful in calming her down in living with him. She states that she also does not have access to her tap dancing which she had to curtail secondary to balance difficulties, and she greatly misses the physical activity and the social component of this.

She states that her appetite is okay, but she estimates that she has lost about 10 pounds over the last few months. Sleep is described as fairly good, though energy level is reported as low.

Psychosocially, the patient was born in Sherwood, North Dakota, first raised for a couple of years in Montana, attended the second grade in Iowa before the family moved to Seattle when she was in the third grade. She is the youngest of 3 raised in an intact family where her father was a barber and mother sewed to help support the family. She attended public schools and was a high school graduate with a high B average, stating that she generally enjoyed school except for one subject that she could not remember. She stated that because of it being the depression time, there were no funds for her to go to college.

The patient has been married to her husband, Walter, since she was 22. She has 3 children, 2 sons and a daughter. He is retired from management at Pacific Northwest Bell. They have been living in their current home for over 50 years. As noted, there has been more recent stress with her husband. She states that her children are quite supportive and have hired someone 3 days a week, in the afternoon, to help with her husband's ADLs (activities of daily living).

Behaviorally, Mrs. Marshall presented promptly, nicely groomed and attired in youthful-appearing clothes. She ambulates without any unusual gait pattern in a slow, steady manner. She was entirely comfortable with being separated from her daughter. Conversational speech was grammatically and syntactically intact, nondysarthric, with clear word-finding difficulties. Thought processes were spontaneous and somewhat tangential. Mood and affect appeared mildly dysthymic, nonlabile, and nonirritable.

Separate interview with daughter, Faith, indicates that the patient has been having difficulty with short-term memory and confusion, repeating herself up to 3 times in an hour, not remembering details such as the procedure for today and resulting frustration. Cognitive difficulties have become much more noticeable to the family in the last 6 months. There has been a concern about her driving in terms of remembering the streets. They stated that premorbidly she was always an extremely avid reader with an excellent vocabulary. Initially, the patient's daughter-in-law felt that Mrs. Marshall may have sustained a concussion when she fell approximately a year and a half ago, although the scans were not consistent with that. Thus far, she is still remembering her daughter's cell phone number and calling her regularly. Recently, the patient also wrote a note to Faith that was logical and made sense. She feels that it has clearly been more stressful for the patient since her husband has returned to live with her.

ASSESSMENT PROCEDURE

Mrs. Marshall and her daughter, Faith, are separately interviewed, recently medical chart reviewed, and the following psychological test instruments administered as part of the neuropsychological evaluation: Portions of the Wechsler Adult Intelligence Scale-III; portions of the Wechsler Memory Scale-III; Boston Naming Test; Verbal Fluency Test; Rey Complex Figure; and Trail Making Test.

TEST-TAKING BEHAVIOR

Mrs. Marshall was very humorous, easy to be with, and was friendly and appropriate. While she understood basic language, she had clear word-finding difficulty and demonstrated frustration with some of the memory tests. Her level of effort was reasonable, and the present results are believed to be a valid estimate of her current level of neurocognitive functioning.

ASSESSMENT RESULTS

Mrs. Marshall is currently oriented to person, place, and most aspects of time, though she erred in stating the date, initially in the 1900s and then changed it to 1003. (I suspect that she meant 2003.) On request to draw a clock and set it to the appropriate time, she does a reasonable job without glaring visual-spatial deficits.

With respect to selected aspects of expressive language, she obtains a total score of 45 out of 60 on Boston Naming Test, which places her in the low-average range compared to other people of her age and educational level. She moderately benefited from phonemic cueing indicating that a number of the missed words were previously familiar to her. On a verbal Fluency Test, she generates 32 words across 3 letters, placing her in the average range, again, compared to other people of her age and educational level.

Examination of selected aspects of intellectual functioning yields the following characteristics: Mrs. Marshall is able to correctly repeat 8 digits in the forward direction and 4 in the reverse, indicating very good basic attention and good concentration skills at present (DIGIT SPAN equals 14). Fund of information reflecting acquired educational experiences and verbal abstracting ability within a structured format are both performed in the average range (INFORMATION equals 10; SIMILARITIES equals 10). Social and practical judgment is performed in the above-average range (COMPREHENSION equals 12). Within the performance section, she is demonstrating average visual attention to details and on a visual-spatial problem solving task (PICTURE COMPLETION equals 9; BLOCK DESIGN equals 9). Overall, she appears to be holding her own in terms of selected aspects of intellectual functioning.

Examination of new learning and memory yields the following characteristics: Immediate recall of paragraph length contextual material is performed in the low-average range, with no recall over a time delay of any aspect of the story, considered a mild to moderately impaired performance. Immediate recognition of faces is performed in the low-average range, with solid improvement over a time delay to a performance in the above-average range. Immediate reproduction of relatively simple geometric figures is performed in a moderately impaired range, with no recall over a time delay, considered mildly impaired for her age. On complex visual-spatial memory test, the Rey Complex Figure, her immediate reproduction shows evidence for mild visual-spatial impairments and preservative tendencies. Over time delay, she is unable to recall any aspects of the figure as well. In summary, then, there is evidence for clear retrieval impairments for both verbal as well as visual information.

Speed and flexibility of thinking as reflected on Trail Making Test is significantly compromised, again compared to age norms. She requires 129 seconds to complete part A, making 1 error in the middle connecting the number 4 to 6. When an element of cognitive flexibility is introduced, in part B, she requires 7 minutes 35 seconds to complete the task.

SUMMARY AND IMPRESSION

Mrs. Corrine Marshall is a delightful 87-year-old right-handed, married, high school graduate whose family has been noting some increasing short-term memory difficulty in the last 4 to 6 months. The patient herself Is noting some word-finding difficulty and some momentary confusion while driving locally in her community, in terms of findings the streets. There has been significant psychosocial stress in this time frame with the advent of her verbally abusive husband moving back into the family home this past Christmas due to insufficient funds to maintain him in a nursing home. The patient continues to remain independent in taking her medications as well as with some limited cooking, although she states that she has never been a good cook. Her older son has taken over managing the bills and has power of attorney.

Recent SPECT scan reveals a large area of decreased activity in the posterior left frontal lobe, a small area of decreased activity in the inferior posterior right frontal lobe, and decreased activity in the right thalamus.

The current neuropsychological test findings show a pattern of mild-to-moderate neurocognitive difficulties in a somewhat diffuse pattern. In addition to clear word-finding difficulties, Mrs. Marshall is demonstrating clear impairments in the acquisition and retrieval of new information of both a visual as well as verbal nature. Speed and flexibility of thinking is compromised, and she is demonstrating mild visual-spatial impairments, suggesting right hemispheric inefficiencies consistent with parietal lobe dysfunction. At the same time, she is demonstrating a number of strengths, including good basic attention and concentration skills, good verbal fluency, and relative preservation of intellectual ability, particularly verbally-mediated crystallized intelligence. Social and practical judgment at the present is good.

While the patient acknowledges that she has been resentful of her need to care for her husband and frustrated by her cognitive diff, an exclusively functional explanation for the current pattern of neurocognitive difficulties is not compelling. This presentation is not suggestive of a circumscribed aphasia, but rather of the beginning stages of a dementia. Given that, I think it was extremely appropriate of Mrs. Marshall to assign financial responsibilities and power of attorney to one of her children. I think that the time is coming close for her to refrain from driving, although I know that this is going to be extremely difficult for her given her need for some break and freedom from her husband. I think that the family might want to consider whether the couple would be best served with some increased assistance in the home, including helping Mrs. Marshall getting out for some needed breaks. Alternatively, they may want to look into an assisted living situation for the couple, as I suspect their needs are going to only increase with time.

Finally, I think that it would be very reasonable for Mrs. Marshall to consider a trial of Aricept to help her maintain function as best as possible. I think she can also benefit from a speech and language evaluation to enhance word-finding compensatory strategies as well as develop memory compensations.

Thank you for the opportunity to consult on Mrs. Marshall. I would be more than happy to go over the results of this evaluation, although I understand from her daughter, Faith, that you will do this at your next appointment. A total of six hours was spent in interviewing Mrs. Marshall and her daughter, administering psychological tests, scoring and interpreting tests, and dictating this report.

Anonymous Ph.D., A.B.P.P.

CPSIA information can be obtained
at www.ICGtesting.com
Printed in the USA
FSHW011323030119
54816FS

9 781721 171149